W9-AQF-108

Watts School of Nursing Library
D.C.H.C.

ON DEATH WITHOUT DIGNITY
The Human Impact of Technological Dying

PERSPECTIVES ON DEATH AND DYING Series
RICHARD A. KALISH, Series Editor

DAVID WENDELL MOLLER

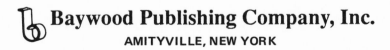 Baywood Publishing Company, Inc.
AMITYVILLE, NEW YORK

10072

As
measured notes
of set music
we pass
in fast or slow
marches
to the grave

Anonymous Tombstone

Watts School of Nursing Library
D.C.H.C.

Copyright © 1990 by the Baywood Publishing Company, Inc., Amityville, New York. All rights reserved. Printed in the United States of America.

Library of Congress Catalog Number: 90-1178
ISBN: 0-89503-066-7 (Paper)
ISBN: 0-89503-067-5 (Cloth)

Library of Congress Cataloging-in-Publication Data

Moller, David Wendell.
   On death without dignity : the human impact of technological dying
   / David Wendell Moller.
        p.   cm.   – –   (Perspectives on death and dying series ;   6)
   Includes bibliographical references and index.
   ISBN   0-89503-066-7   (paper).   – –   ISBN   0-89503-067-5   (cloth)
   1. Thanatology.   2. Death—Social aspects.   3. Terminal care–
   –United States.   I. Title.   II. Series.
   HQ1073.5.U6M65   1990
   306.9—dc20   90-1178

HQ
1073.5
.U6
M7260
1990

In memory of my mother
Frances Wendell Moller
who showed me the value of knowledge,
and from whom I learned that the
tribulations of suffering can lead to
the joy of life.

For my father
William Moller
in deepest thanks
for his continuous support and understanding.

And
In memory of the lives and suffering of the
dying people without whom this book
would not have been possible.

Preface

One indispensable measure of the human condition is the way in which humanity responds to suffering, tragedy, and death. Dying, which is the focus of this book, is not just a medically and personally relevant process. It is a part of human life which has tremendous symbolic significance. It symbolizes the meaning of the collective fate of human beings, namely, our mortality. Moreover, it symbolizes the presence of dreaded qualities of human existence: loneliness, pain, untold suffering, deterioration, helplessness and meaninglessness. The symbolization of dying in modern American society is permeated with threatening and catastrophic images. Clearly, by studying dying and its cultural symbols or meanings much is learned about human responses to mortality. More importantly, the study of dying unveils much about the nature of human life. Ironically, one of the most instructive ways to learn about human living is to study human dying and death. The folkways of dying and death are a mirror which reflects the folkways, values, meanings, and patterns of living. Consequently, the ways, means, and meanings of dying are indicative of the ways, means, and meanings of living.

At its very simplest, the quality of dying is a reflection of the quality of living; a measure of the condition of human life. On a deeper level, dying and death are indicators of perplexing and complex, psychological and social issues that typify a given cultural context. Efforts to understand the personal and social factors of dying provide insight into the viability of cultural values, social institutions, and patterns of human behavior in ameliorating the plight of dying individuals. Perhaps one of the best tests of the quality and meaning of prevailing patterns of living is the way in which these patterns influence and shape the course of human dying. For these reasons, this book is not just about human dying, it is about life and living as well.

Studying the context and circumstances of dying and how these circumstances facilitate or hinder the development of human or social qualities relevant to meaning, purpose and well-being is potentially liberating and freeing. On a personal level, dying and death are penultimate issues of existential significance. The fact of mortality is one of the most awesome and challenging dimensions of human life. The process of making feasible and workable adjustments to the human fact of finitude is enhanced by coming to grips with the patterns and issues that define the contemporary dying process. Coming to terms with dying and death intellectually facilitates a seedbed of knowledge that enables individuals to make an investment in greater autonomy and self-determination. If used judiciously, the sociomedical study of human dying is potentially emancipating. Through knowledge and understanding, it can aid in facing the prospect of dying with greater purpose and mastery. Scholarly analysis and criticism, whether it be sociological, psychological, sociomedical or otherwise, is an important form of empowerment. The knowledge, understanding, and insight which are the cornerstone of academic inquiry enable individuals and societies to design personal and social systems of living that are creative, constructive and meaningful. This is precisely the spirit in which social criticism is used throughout this book, namely, to endorse and empower the development of patterns of living which nurture the quality of human life, both on a personal and social basis.

There is another important reason for this book, one which is most personally and professionally significant to me. There is no doubt that the dying patients who participated in this study were the greatest teachers about life that I have ever had. Their experiences, especially their suffering, often went unrecognized and their lives were all too often jeopardized by isolation. This book is an attempt to tell part of their story. It is an attempt to bring their suffering and tribulations out of the deep freeze of isolation and silence, where most Americans prefer to keep such unappealing topics. Thus, while I am speaking in a scholarly framework, more importantly, I am speaking for the dying patients who shared their deepest frailties, anxieties, and vulnerabilities in a way that expressed the zenith of courage. Their story, all the more urgent for it typically not being told, is an important story. They and other patients who are now or will someday be in their place deserve to have their plight expressed with candor and sensitivity. If I have succeeded in this task, perhaps some value will be derived from their suffering, dying and deaths.

My deepest gratitude is extended to these patients. Not only have they made this study possible, they have enriched my life personally and professionally.

My intellectual debt for this book is considerable. My passion for learning was initiated by the Christian Brothers of La Salle Military Academy. Richard Connors provided continuous personal and intellectual challenge during my formative intellectual years. I thank him for his love, support and perspicacity. Merle Longwood introduced me to the importance of sociomedical and bioethical issues as fields of scholarly study. My academic interest in death and dying is directly traceable to his teaching and research endeavors. Dennis O'Connor, one of the greatest teachers I have ever had, showed me that intellectual activity can be one of life's most satisfying passions. Barry Pehrsson introduced me to critical sociological perspectives and was instrumental in nurturing my critical, intellectual sensibilities.

My early years of graduate training at the New School for Social Research introduced me to the exciting world of sociological theory in a way that was unique and inspiring. Special thanks are owed to David Muchnick, Arthur Vidich and Stanford Lyman.

My doctoral training at Columbia University provided access to some of the finest sociomedical scholars in the world. My debt to John Colombotos is unmeasurable and unpayable. He is a teacher and mentor par excellence. His support, scholarly leadership, and continual guidance were seminal forces in my academic development. The Foundation of Thanatology provided continuing support and encouragement for this project. I am also indebted to Mitch Schorow, Austin Kutscher and Allan Barton, who played various roles in helping me develop the research study which resulted in this book. My debt to Bob DeBellis is immeasurable.

Richard Kalish has been supportive and constructive in his criticism of this work. He was excited about the publication of the book and was writing an Afterword for it. Unfortunately, his untimely death made it impossible for his insights to appear in these pages.

Jack Elinson has had a major impact on my scholarly development during my years of training at Columbia. I am honored that he has written the Introductory Précis to this book.

My colleagues at Indiana University have been continuing sources of support and encouragement. I would like to particularly express my thanks to Linda Haas, John Liell, David Ford, Ain Haas, and Morris Weinberger. John Barlow and Bill Plater have been exceptionally supportive of this project.

A special debt of gratitude is owed to Robert Anderson, who always had faith in my intellectual potential. I thank him for his support and for the many hours we have spent in intellectual interchange. Regina Kenen has been a source of support and advocacy since the early stages of my career. Her faith in me is one of the rarest gifts a young scholar can receive.

I thank Susan Engel and Barbara Bogue, my research assistants, for their support, hard work, and friendship during the preparation of this manuscript. The future of academic activity in America is bright with young intellectual talent such as theirs to meaningfully respond to the demands and responsibilities of intellectual life. I thank Kathy Benoit for her assistance in typing this manuscript. Special thanks go to Amy van der Vliet.

My wife, Mary, has been a constant source of support during the preparation of this book. Her love, understanding, and nurturance have had an unparalleled impact on my life. In many ways, this impact is present throughout these pages.

The strengths and virtues of this book are a direct result of the dedication of the above individuals, as people and as professionals. The weaknesses of the book are my responsibility, and mine alone.

It was Camus and Dostoyevsky who advanced the theme that the path to joy leads through suffering. While this book is clearly about human suffering, I hasten to emphasize that my study and observations are driven by a love of and respect for life, not a morbid or depressing obsession with death and suffering. It may very well be that on a personal and societal level, the folkways of dying are the richest representation of human self-expresssion. It may very well be that the ways in which human beings face up to the mystery that is the end of life is the final and greatest statement about the value and meaning of life itself. In this way, candid awareness and understanding of the situation of modern dying people are essential to understanding the pathways to joy and the means of achieving authenticity in living. When you hear the words of the dying people throughout the pages of this book, they are expressing two very important messages. One has to do with the horribleness of the modern experience of dying and death; the other loudly affirms the sweetness and essential goodness of living. Thus, this study of death is a study of life that is deeply enmeshed in a belief in the value and potential of all human existence. And it is by journeying through suffering, such as illustrated in the chapters to follow, that the splendor of living can be fully unveiled.

David Wendell Moller, Ph.D.
Indianapolis, Indiana

Précis

"Are you dying?" . . . "Why? Can't you see I am?" . . . "Well, get on with
your dying; don't raise a blamed fuss over that job. We can't help you"
[1, p. 331].

Joseph Conrad

In the 20th century rush to technologize medicine, the hospital has become an
inappropriate place to die. The earlier fear of hospitals as the place where poor
people went to die has been overcome. Most people admitted to hospitals are
now discharged alive. Thanks to biomedical inventiveness a few remain dying
for a long time. When the brain ceases to function, the heart muscle can be kept
beating. Quaternary care has become awesome.

Caught up with new medical knowledge—mostly, with halfway technologies—
physicians, always uncomfortable with failure, are more reluctant than ever to
give up. Technologies are applied beyond reasonable expectations that patients
can be restored to functioning human beings. So long as the heart muscle can be
kept beating, there is a wish, almost unconscious, that the body ensemble will
achieve a recognizable living condition. Who knows? Tomorrow a new biomedical discovery may bring the patient around.

Yet, even as more and more people die in the hospital, it is less and less considered to be an appropriate place to die. Other institutions, called hospices,
have sprung up to better serve the dying. Hospices are not yet so plentiful, however, that they can take over the dying from the hospitals. Physicians in hospitals
are dedicated to the prevention of dying. Physicians do not define themselves as
ministering to the dying. So long as physicians maintain their authority in hospitals, dying patients will be kept from death by available technology.

Yet dying patients do eventually die; and for some this may take a long time.
How does the hospital, particularly the attending physician, deal with this? Not
very well, according to sociologist David Moller. Applying a sociomedical perspective to complement the biomedical perspectives of hospital physicians, Moller critically examines medical folkways in the hospital with respect to dying.
He finds that physicians see no purpose in dying. He argues that if we understood
more about dying we would gain in our power to "design personal and social
systems of living, that are creative, constructive and meaningful." By way of the
intensive, scholarly study he reports here, Moller has become an advocate of
the dying, seeking to reduce their socially enforced isolation.

Dying is not only rejected by hospital physicians as a condition they feel prepared to deal with professionally, but is also neglected in the larger social sphere. How does society respond? Dying is avoided as a subject for conversation. Attention is directed to doing physically possible things. We are lacking in socially acceptable routines in dealing with dying. There are no standards, guidelines or codes. The subject is suppressed as being too depressing. It becomes a totally private phenomenon with which few of us are prepared to deal. Technological concerns displace or, at least, dampen social and emotional involvement. Dying is a reflection on the failure of technology; and modern medicine is nothing if not technology.

Lest he be misunderstood as attacking how physicians respond to dying, Moller does not single out modern medicine as unique or even peculiar in its technological orientation. Rather, he places it in the broader society with its technological emphasis. Technologizing is one of two major social forces which has led to the isolating and falsely hopeful experience of the dying. The second is the cultural value of individualism as manifested in the human potential movement. These two powerful and pervasive social forces are merged in the managing, packaging, and containment of dying as an individual experience subject to unrealistically indefinite, technological postponement. The dying role decimates individual dignity and identity, converting the individual to the "low status of a second-class citizen."

Moller calls for a more candid, open approach to dying which will recognize dying as a normal, social phenomenon as well as a deeply personal, individual experience. He counsels us to abandon technologic intimations of immortality. The creative efforts of individuals, heroic and moving as they may be when confronting dying, need to be buttressed by social legitimation in the form of "prescribed societal rituals, folkways and meaning sets." Individuals and their social networks should not be left entirely to their own resources in coping with dying. Moller wants social recognition of the meanness of dying, especially oncological dying in the hospital, the subject of his empirical observations, with its "experiences of alienation, stigma, helplessness, pain, suffering, normlessness and turbulence."

The current societal approach to dying is silent avoidance. Cultural variation in funeral arrangements is a social response to the actual occurrence of death, not to dying. There are no dying "images and themes" in ordinary social intercourse. This is a 20th century phenomenon, unlike preceding centuries. Dying is now shameful, dirty, improper and a social evil since it is outside of technological control. It is disinfected by medicalization in the hospital technocracy. As Glaser and Strauss have shown, the reality of dying is hidden by conspiratorial interaction of doctors, nurses, patients and their families.

Moller identifies de-humanization of medical care as a structural force, rooted in the way physicians are trained and perpetuated by the peer culture and organization of medical work. With Renée Fox he recognizes the importance of the human anatomy laboratory with its cadavers as the place where medical students learn detached concern, even callousness. In the case of the dying, physician's priorities are activities which medically benefit patients. When doctors note that death is imminent, Moller observed "a formal and regular rush to move on to the next patient and on to another floor." He concludes that there is increasing normlesness with respect to how physicians should relate to dying patients. As medical technology becomes more rational, more uncertainty is introduced into interactions between physicians and dying patients, leaving this to individual physicians and patients.

The ultimate powerlessness of the dying is reflected in the behavior not only of the patient, but also in that of the physician and the hospital. Family and friends are limited in their experience with dying as a social phenomenon. Society has as yet failed to provide the necessary rules for processing the inevitable ultimate failure of science and technology to prevent what is after all a universal social as well as biological event.

Moller is not content with phenomenological description and analysis. He further provides us not only with social diagnosis, but also calls for social prescriptions. Social rules and behavior need to be invented for the social phenomenon of oncological dying and put into practice in order to respond to:

- the sense of isolation of dying patients and loved ones
- the feelings of powerlessness of dying patients and loved ones
- the devaluation of the dying experience
- the downward path of pain, suffering and deterioration experienced by the dying person
- the stigma of dying
- the hopelessness, helplessness, ugliness, anxiety and frustration of the dying process
- the unrelieved pain of oncological dying
- the feelings of vulnerability when emotional and social needs are inadequately met
- the feelings of self-blame, guilt and dependency
- the feelings of rejection as a sexual being
- undignified dying patient behavior, such as anger, cantankerousness, and behavioral expression of private, negative feelings
- romantic, sentimental, and overly-inflated expressions of grief.

Such social rules and behavior could, according to Moller:

- re-introduce a peaceful sense of harmony between dying people and the process of dying
- provide the support of community participation in dying rituals
- be a force for the harmonious acceptance of the coming of death as an ordinary and natural process as opposed to a social evil

- emphasize the comforting roles of fellowship, ritual, and ceremony
- facilitate, even mandate, the notion that dying should be a culturally shared community experience
- culturally legitimate the pain and suffering that often typifies the experience of dying
- provide a common base of participation and sense of belonging; attach the dying person to the community of living.

This prescriptive catalogue of social rules and behavior could, in David Moller's view, transform and retrieve the process of dying from a medicalized technology to a natural social experience. As plausible and rational as his analysis, diagnosis and prescription seem, it remains to be seen how compliant society will be. In any case, he has vividly reminded us that dying is a social phenomenon as well as an individual event; and that attention to its social components may provide us with social dignity when faced with an inevitable biological occurrence.

REFERENCE

1. J. Conrad, The Nigger of Narcissus in *The Portable Conrad,* Revised Edition, M. D. Zabel (ed.), Penguin Books, New York, 1977.

Jack Elinson

Table of Contents

Introduction

There is no love of life without despair of life. [1, p. 56]

Albert Camus

A man in his mid-fifties sat on the edge of his hospital bed, holding on to his IV pole. He had extensive involvement of cancer in his kidneys, and his vanishing healthy cell tissue was rapidly being replaced by the accumulation of water in the abdominal area. The twenty or twenty-five pounds of fluid which had accumulated in his stomach provided an absurd counterbalancing image to his otherwise frail frame. The oncologist walked into the patient's room, in mid-afternoon, finding him disoriented, slightly hallucinatory, in danger of falling out of bed and toppling over onto his IV connection and, very much alone. The bed-tray had been pushed to one corner of the room, where it rested with medicines that were not administered and with food that had not been eaten.

When the oncologist returned later that evening, the man's wife had come to visit him, after work. The patient was lying securely in his bed, but his bed-tray was still full with uneaten food and unadministered medicine. The doctor began talking to the man's wife, telling her that her husband would not be released over the weekend. He told her that she simply would not be able to manage him at home, so it would be best if he stayed where he was. He also commented that they would have to wait and see how he was progressing, and then begin to think about letting him go home during the middle of the following week. (The physician, however, had fully anticipated that this patient would die sometime over the weekend, if not that very night.) He also expressed his belief that the patient should have someone attend him, round the clock. While voicing some concern over whether or not this could be managed financially, he felt it would be best for the patient's safety, given his worry about the patient's disorientation and newly developed inclination to try to get out of bed. The patient's wife responded that if it needed to be done, she would go ahead and make the necessary arrangements with the hospital cashier. The oncologist informed the wife that one of his associates would be making rounds over the weekend and he wished her good night.

The physician, upon leaving the patient's room, summoned one of the floor nurses and gave her verbal instructions (which were also appropriately written into the patient's chart) on what needed to be done for the patient, including making sure that his medications were fully administered.

1

In this brief case example, there are many ordinary processes, related to modern dying, that are taking place. There are no medical heroics involved, there is no extraordinary machinery in place, and the patient was admitted onto a general medical floor. In a certain sense, the situation of this dying patient is quite normative and typically found in modern hospital settings. The patient had been treated for his disease for nine months, had been in and out of the hospital several times, was still within a framework of active chemotherapy for his cancer, and was receiving medical treatment for the physical symptoms that occurred from his disease. At this point, the patient was basically in an "auto-pilot" situation, a medical holding pattern, where his symptoms would be actively treated, and a wait-and-see attitude developed on whether he would live for days, a week, a month or die very soon.

Death, of course, is present in this holding pattern, but then again it is very much absent. In terms of interaction with the patient and his wife, the idea or possibility of death—not to mention the reality that the patient was dying—was never discussed. Indeed, dying was isolated from conversations that took place, and conversations which took place isolated dying from the context of verbal interaction. It was clear, however, that the issue of dying was very much in the heart, mind and tearful eyes of the patient's wife. However, the physician directed the course of interaction away from dying as he steered concern toward practical, technical, medical matters. In this way, dying becomes very difficult to detect; it is disguised as the need for physical management and symptom treatment, and thereby is excluded from the regular, ongoing flow of doctor-patient, doctor-family interaction.

The absence of guidelines or moral codes to direct the behaviors of those involved in the human experience of dying leaves the participants with a feeling of not knowing what to say or what to do. Adopting a line of response that emphasizes the management of physical needs is consistent with the training and work orientation of the profession of medicine. The physician, in this frame of reference which transforms the human dying experience into a series of physical treatment endeavors, is enabled to work in a setting where dying abounds without having to confront the emotional and social issues that form the human process of dying and death. The issue of dying is thereby isolated in the private experiences and world view of patients and families. While patients and their loved ones are understandably concerned with the overriding question, "Is this dying or death?," the issue of dying is not an acceptable basis for conversations and interactions with physicians. Thus, patients, families and physicians approach the experience of dying from sharply divergent perspectives. The former emphasizes the personal and social implications of dying, whereas physicians adopt a preeminently technical approach to their relationship with dying patients.

It is this pattern of interaction, that invokes a deafening silence about dying and death, which is a penultimate source of social isolation for the dying patient.

The emotional neutrality and objective-technical emphasis of the medical care-takers facilitate the isolation of emotional and social needs of dying patients. This leads patients into a private, personal, isolated, and encapsulated world. In this way, one of the major consequences of the technological management of the process of dying is the containment of the human experiences of dying in the private territory of dying patients and their intimates.

The theme of managing the experience of human dying through technological manipulation of the dying process and through the social isolation of individual dying patients is central to this book. I will explore how the American value of individualism and commitment to technology have given rise to particular forms of controlling the process of dying in the hospital setting. I will focus attention on how the values of technology in the broader society are applied in the framework of medicalized care of the dying patient and on the consequences this has for the lives of dying patients. Additionally, I will analyze how the value of individualism, so ubiquitous in the broader society, influences the treatment of dying patients and their definition of the situation of their own dying. In this way, I will show how some of the values of the American cultural system are institutionalized in the medical treatment of dying patients, and how internalization of the values of the broader American culture, along with the institutionalization of medicalized dying, shape the experience of dying for individual patients.

My explicit purpose in this book is to analyze dying and death in the cosmopolitan, modern setting. There is, however, an additional subject that is implicitly addressed in my analysis and observations. The portrait of dying which is provided in the pages to follow also shows us a great deal about the nature of life in latter-day, twentieth-century America. As emphasized in the Preface, the styles and patterns of dying and death are reflective of the styles and patterns of life in a particular historical and cultural circumstance. Indeed, the more I study in and learn about the field of death and dying, the more I am convinced that *the way one dies is a reflection of the way one lives*. This is not just relevant for the personal, private lives of individuals. It is also appropriate on a societal level. In particular, the circumstances of an individual's private life—the quality of relationships, spirituality, personality characteristics, etc.— are significant to the unique way each person will endure his or her own dying experience. More broadly, the dominant patterns of life and socialization in the larger society will significantly shape and define the contours of the collective dying experience in American society. Thus, by understanding the nature of human dying in American society, an important insight is gained into the patterns of living in America.

It is precisely for these reasons that the study of dying and death, which on the surface appears to be morbid, can be one of the deepest pronouncements of the love of life. The questions which are raised by the study of dying and death are questions that are seminal to the study of life. Issues such as the meaning of life and death, the meaning and the impact of suffering, and the value of social support and intimacy are not just narrowly related to death and dying. They are major issues defining the patterns of life in America today. The study of the suffering, agony, dilemmas, pain, and terror of dying is useful for generating explanations and understandings which have the potential for ameliorating the *life* circumstances of dying patients. Just as importantly, this study provides insights on how the human quest for meaning, satisfaction and joy in living, is being satisfied on a daily basis for all citizens. By approaching the study of dying as a cultural and structural reflection of living, one can generate insights into both dying and living which are sensitive to the affirmation of the goodness and value of life for all human beings—healthy, disabled, sick, or dying. If there was one dominant unspoken message which I read in the eyes of the dying patients whose lives and sufferings so enrich this book, it ran something like this: "Tell your students, your readers that despite the incomprehensibility of our sufferings, this is truth not fiction. Revel in the joy and goodness of life. For as we, the dying, thirst for health, normalcy and a future, those of you with all of these gifts at your doorstep, owe it to us not to take life and its splendor for granted. Appreciate each breath that you draw, for someday soon, each of us is going to be dead for an awfully long time." The most important message of these dying patients was not about death. It was about life.

This book, with the landscape of modern dying which it portrays, is dedicated to the lives and sufferings of all dying human beings—both present and future.

REFERENCE

1. A. Camus, *Lyrical and Critical Essays,* Random House, New York, 1968.

CHAPTER
1

Technology, Meaning and Death

How the tumor was spreading! Seen through the eyes of a complete stranger it would be frightening enough, but seen through his own . . .! No, this thing could not be real. No one else around him had anything like it. In all his forty-five years Pavel Nikolayevich had never seen such a deformity . . . [1, p. 18]

"If only it would stop growing!" said Pavel Nikolayevich, as though begging it to stop. His voice was tearful. "If only it would stop! If it goes on growing like this for another week, Goodness only knows. . . ." No, he couldn't say it, he couldn't gaze into the black abyss. How miserable he felt—it was all touch-and-go. "The next injection's tomorrow, then one on Wednesday. But what if it doesn't do any good? What shall I do?" [1, p. 176]

Alexander Solzhenitsyn

Science and technology assume a panacea-like character; given only time, the fantasy is that all problems will capitulate to it. Man is really a Promethean and there is presumably nothing he cannot accomplish [2, pp. 260–261].

Alvin Gouldner

As one surveys the values, institutions, and people of America, it is not difficult to see the centrality of science and technology to the economic and social forces of society. In many ways the combined scientific and technological efforts of the private and public sector are so vast that they are beyond the comprehension of ordinary citizens. Yet, technology has become so consistently and deeply a part of everyday life that American people have fallen rather blindly in love with it [3, p. 34], albeit if in a take-it-for-granted way. As Edward Shils observes, Americans have fully committed themselves to a scientific way of life even without concrete guarantees and evidence that science improves upon the quality of life:

. . . readiness to support science rests in part on the belief that science contributes to the material well-being of society. . . . At present, the evidence that fundamental scientific research contributes to material well-being is very uneven and not by any means vigorously conclusive. The

5

conclusion is accepted because there is a mood to accept it. . . . But it is largely a matter of faith . . . and derived from a profound and diffuse "will to believe" in the efficacy of science [4, p. 3].

This faith in science reflects an underlying attitude of the American people; a sensibility which inherently values science and its ways of life. Consistent with the conviction that science improves the livability of life is the belief that technological by-products of scientific activity make life more meaningful and facilitate the improvement of personal and social problems [5, Chapters 2-5]. While it may be overstating the current course of affairs to suggest, as Ellul [6] and others have, that America is exclusively dominated by technical forces, it is not pressing too far to note that recent decades of American life have given rise to a sustained and national commitment to a scientific and technological orientation.

Some scholars would have us believe that technology is ethically neutral, that is to say, that once having been created, it does not possess self-sustaining life or momentum of its own but rather is used for purposes good or bad by humanity. While I do not necessarily disagree with these utopian scholars who see technology as a tool in the hands of humanity, there is mounting evidence that the presence of the tool has an inevitable and significant impact on the tool holder. In addition, the philosophy which surrounds and has been internalized by the tool holder, a philosophy which promotes the value of tools in particular and the process of tool making in general, has an intractable value-relevant impact on the men and women who use the products of science and technology in their daily lives. Thus, while humanity may not be inescapably imprisoned by technological forces, the role of technology in modern society is so pervasive that individuals cannot avoid being influenced and directed by the social forces which associate with technology and its development.

The work of Gouldner is seminal in addressing this issue of the impact of technology on the social conditions of human life. In *The Dialectic of Ideology and Technology*, Gouldner discusses the transformation of traditional, ritual-based, religious society into systems of thought and activity which are more secular:

> The rise and development of modern ideologies was shaped by the rise of modern science, by the growing prestige of technology and new modes of production, and by the development of publics whose favorable judgment of modern science was rooted in the decline of older authority-referencing discourse. Science became the prestigious and focally visible paradigm of the new mode of discourse; it was this mode of discourse, which diffuses the seen-but-unnoticed set of background assumptions, on which science itself was tacitly grounded [2, p. 7].

The connection between science and technology and value-laden ideology is carefully unveiled by Gouldner's analysis. The inescapable paradox of science, and even of the social sciences, with their pretense to value-neutrality, is that it embraces the values of rationality and efficiency in its quest for objectivity.

Thus, as society modernized, that is to say moved toward the grounding of action in rational and secular thought, traditional world views of myth, religion, and metaphysics were systematically devalued. New legitimations appeared in the mantle of science, and were affirmed by the modernizing citizenry. In this way, from its origin, science is not value-free but is carried out within a framework that values the scientific mode of living. Science and technology have become a dominant, value based ideology of society with which, in one way or another, humanity has to come to terms.

In an important way, the American scientific and technological orientation affects the symbols and the values to and through which people relate to society and society "relates" to people. For example, as the power of traditional systems of authority declined and was supplanted by the growth of rationalization of thought, one of the primary underlying catalysts of the growth of the rational orientation was the development of the technology of printing. As printing became more and more widespread, explanations for human and social living were no longer exclusively linked to sacred and unquestionable definitions of the world. The idea of rational discourse, the intellectual clash between competing and often contradicting interpretations of reality, became increasingly relevant for society. But the age of rationality presumed literacy and hence elicited the development, spread, and organization of printing. This, in turn, produced a growing supply of pamphlets, newsletters, newspapers, books, and journals that were partly a response to and partly a source of growing literacy [2, p. 40].

The relevant point is twofold: 1) the revolution of printing technology was grounded in a culture of growing scientism, and; 2) the technology of printing had an important impact on shaping the social character structure of human personality. The following discussion illustrates one of the major consequences of this technological-social change for human personality.

Prior to printing, human communication primarily occurred in a social context among human aggregates: people talking face to face with others. Communication was inherently a collectivizing social phenomenon. However, the printed word began another tradition, one of the isolation of human communication. As Neil Postman comments, with the printed book came the isolated reader and his private eye. In this sense, reading and printing technology represented a conspiracy against human community and social presence [7, p. 27]. Indeed, as Gouldner suggests, printing does allow for separation of talk from the talker [2, p. 41], but more importantly allows for a single individual to speak to large numbers of distinct and unrelated individuals in the absence of a shared social context. Additionally, the more contemporary development of electronic media technology (radio, television) has made the separation of physical proximity and social interaction-communication all the more widespread and accessible [8, pp. 116–118].

Thus, printing technology initiated the mass media movement which introduced into society the social categories of public and mass society. But the irony of this is that the existence of a public requires people to be treated as private persons [2, p. 98]. In the framework I have briefly delineated here, one can see how the modernization of society has entailed the transformation of once isolated individuals into a public while simultaneously keeping the public isolated individuals. The massification of modern-technical society then was predicated on the privatization of the individual and the technological revolution of European society inherently gave rise to the burgeoning of individualism [9].

I have selectively sketched the association between technology and individualism in the modern society to stress that the progress of modern civilization itself was and is largely defined by these social forces. Indeed, the technological foundation of society in large part facilitates the excessive individualism, detached egoism, and absence of shared concerns which characterize our age [10, 11]. It is also these social forces of technology and individualism, inherent to the modern American way of life, which are pre-eminent factors in shaping and defining the experience of dying and death for modern individuals.

MEANING OF DEATH OR DEATH OF MEANING

The scientific orientation of American society is closely linked with the value of materialism. In other words, science has merged with technology and technology has become science-based [12]. The core motivational ideology of society lies within this framework of the fusion of science and technology. But yet, the scientific and technological orientation is a dominant force in society, not just in an ethereal-ideological way, but as part of a concrete, pragmatic program of social progress and personal betterment. The technological consciousness of modern American society sees science and technology as a utopian absolute, integrating good intentions with unlimited possibilities, in the pursuit of the elimination of social evils [2, Chapter 12; 5, Chapter 2]. However, the technocratic consciousness becomes meaningfully relevant to the everyday life of ordinary citizens through the value of materialism, and the loyalty of ordinary citizens is cemented to the technocratic system through technologically based gratifications, that is to say, "consumerism" [2, p. 262].

The degree to which the technocratic way of life is adopted by society and its people, the definition of personal and social worth becomes characterized by the equation, I AM = WHAT I HAVE AND WHAT I CONSUME [13, p. 15]. More importantly, within a framework where the value of life is defined through possessions and materialism, death and dying represent penultimate threats to the utopian vision of the technocratic world view. Dying and death threaten to deprive one of security, of identity, of those qualities which provide modern individuals with a sense of self-importance and social status. Thus, as long as the technocratic way of life and definition of reality prevail, dying and death must be feared. Erich Fromm effectively articulates the point:

> There is only one way—taught by the Budda, by Jesus, by the Stoics, by Master Eckhart—to truly overcome the fear of dying, and that way

is by *not hanging onto life, not experiencing life as a possession.* . . .
The fear, then, is not of dying, but of losing WHAT I HAVE: The fear
of losing my body, my ego, my possessions, and my identity; the fear
of facing the abyss of nonidentity of "being lost."

To the extent that we live in the having mode, we must fear dying
[13, p. 112].

Dying is intolerable to the technocratic consciousness since it blemishes
the technical ideals of omnipotence and abundance, with scarcity and vulnerability. Dying points out the weaknesses of the technological and scientific lifestyle. Literally dying, especially from cancer, means encroaching
helplessness, physical deterioration, alienation, emotional turbulence, and
of course, makes the pursuit of materialism empty and moot. The major societal response to the intolerable social evil of dying is technological intervention. As we shall see in subsequent chapters, it is the technological orientation
of society in general and of the profession of medicine in particular which is
unable to provide for legitimation, purpose, and meaning to the dying experience. Consequently, an antagonistic relationship between technocratic consciousness and dying is spawned and the ultimate goal of the technological
management of dying becomes the defeat of death.

I do not mean to imply that the technocratic coordination of society and
the technical management of death have marched forward without resistance.
In recent decades the counter-cultural movement of the sixties and the inva-
sion of the theme of 'hi-touch' in the seventies and eighties has sought to bring
something seemingly non-technical to the technological orientation of modern
social living. Indeed, one response to the growth of the technical system was the
emergence of a highly individualized, personal value system to compensate for
the impersonal nature of technology. The result was the new self-help or personal growth movement [14, p. 36]. As we have already seen, individualism is
historically consistent and compatible with the technological framework of
modern civilization. It is therefore logical that resistance to an increasingly technocratic style of living would assume the character of individual self-expression
and development. It is in this way that the 'hi-touch' movement pursues qualities that reflect the non-technical and non-mechanical side of life but are also
harmonious with the broader values and framework of technological society.

The human potential movement is not representative of a fundamental
change in the sensibilities of the American culture and its people. This is precisely why the self-growth movement is accepted and even enhanced by the
technocratic consciousness. The nature of self-expression and growth, in the contemporary social setting, is consistent with the HAVING ORIENTATION of the
broader technocratic society. The self in the human potential movement is one's
most precious and important possession. In the HAVING mode, the quintessen-
tial qualities to pursue and achieve are those which enhance and improve the
self. In this way, the self becomes a package to be managed and styled in a
fashion that makes one more cultured, attractive, personable, confident, energetic,

etc. The irony of the course of the development of the self-awareness movement is that at the same time the American individual is becoming increasingly detached from the social bonds of shared concerns and community, the self remains embodied in and connected to ways of living that are products of our common technocratic consciousness.

In the framework of self-growth and expression, scarcity is defined as the presence of factors which threaten to annihilate the self. Of course, death may be seen as the ultimate force of annihilation, but perhaps even more meaningful to the proponents of the human potential movement is the process of dying. If dying obliterates the dignity of the self, the societal movement toward total development of human potential is thwarted. If, on the other hand, ways can be devised to transform the experience of dying into a process of growth, dignity and enrichment, a final triumph—a final victory—is amassed for the self. In a context which views the self as a package or product to be managed and improved, dying can be perceived as an opportunity to embark upon a final management effort ("a final stage of growth"), which asserts the primary value of self and individual development. The emergence of the hospice philosophy, the widespread popularity of Elisabeth Kübler-Ross and Shanti-Nilaya, the recent media attention directed toward death-with-dignity, and the proliferation of little recipe-type, "how-to-do-it" books on death, dying and grieving are effectively explained by the broader societal commitment to the human potential movement.

The key point to emphasize is that the individual is the primary focus of attention in the human potential movement. The individual through his or her own effort, with or without the assistance of others, embarks upon the course of self-improvement and exaltation. Likewise, it is the dying person individually, with or without the assistance of others, who is ultimately responsible for carving out creative and meaningful ways to die. Meaningful death is hence defined through the effort of individuals, not through the existence of prescribed societal rituals, folkways and meaning sets.

As noted earlier, on a personal and societal level, the way one dies is a reflection of the way one lives. The implications of the values of modern living, especially in relation to technology or materialism, and self-expression or individualism, for human death and dying are most effectively illustrated in the work of Leo Tolstoy. In writing what was essentially a prognostication of things to come, it is haunting how accurately Tolstoy's perceptions, recorded one hundred years ago, capture the spirit and course of the modern dying experience. Specifically, in "The Death of Ivan Ilych," Tolstoy portrays a man who had lived most ordinarily, that is to say, in harmony with the prevailing folkways and behavioral expectations of modern society. When Ivan Ilych comes face to face with sickness, sickness that is not relievable by technical intervention, he embarks upon a self-initiated course of seeking to make some sense out of his predicament. But, as Tolstoy describes, modern ideas and systems of living are essentially incompatible with the idea of dying and death:

> Whether it was morning or evening, Friday or Sunday, made no difference, it was all just the same: the gnawing, unmitigated, agonizing pain, never ceasing for an instant, the consciousness of life inexorably waning but not yet extinguished, the approach of that ever dreaded and hateful Death which was the only reality. . . .
> If only it would come quicker! If only WHAT would come quicker? Death, darkness? . . . No, no! Anything rather than death [15, pp. 139–140]!

Ivan Ilych lived in common ordinary consensus with modern values. Consequently he was poorly equipped to make sense out of his dying. There was little legitimation of the dying experience that could be proffered by the cultural and social systems that surrounded Ilych's life. Yet, his quest to find some purpose to his dying assumed the proportions of an obsession:

> "What is it for?" And he ceased crying, but turning his face to the wall continued to ponder the same question: Why, and for what purpose, is there all this horror? . . .
> He suffered ever the same unceasing agonies and in his lonelinesss pondered always on the same insoluble question: "What is this? Can it be that it is Death?" And the inner voice answered: "Yes, it is Death."
> "Why these sufferings?" And the voice answered, "For no reason—they just are so" [15, pp. 148–149].

Ivan Ilych continues his struggle for meaning in the face of death, but there was nothing within the configuration of his society, nor in the way he lived his life, that could help him understand his plight: "There is no explanation! Agony, death . . . What for" [15, p. 151]?

The 'fiction' of Tolstoy finds itself being played out in the lives of terminally-ill patients on a daily basis. Indeed, a commonly voiced question and frustration among dying patients is: "Why did this have to happen to me? I don't know why this had to happen to me anyway." Of course, a satisfying and comforting answer to this and similar questions is not prominently embodied in the cultural and social systems of modern society. It is for this reason that Ivan Ilych, like terminally-ill patients today, was able to find relief from the incessant terror of death only through his remarkable persistence in self-reflection and his personalized heroic effort.[1] And, for Ivan Ilych, it took right up until the moment of death for him to carve out some sense of meaning for and peace with what had happened to him.

In summary, two dominant, interrelated factors are directing the way of the modern dying process: The technocratic orientation of society which is expressed in technologically based programs of patient care found in the medical system, and the absence of culturally shared and defined meanings to the

[1] Increasingly, there are accounts in the literature of individuals seeking and finding a sense of meaning to their cancer/dying experiences. One must remember, however, that meaning is sought in a self-expressive modality, in distinct individual cases, without the regularized support of a commonly shared set of cultural and social systems of legitimation.

experience of dying. As this book will portray, these are two salient forces affecting the lives of dying patients, particularly those majority of patients who die in the technocratic-hospital setting. In this way, the modern dying process is technologically complex but lacks a sense of cosmic connection, lacks involvement with the stable, ongoing community and social rituals, and largely leaves the individual to his or her own resources in coping with the realities of dying. It will be essential to keep the foundation set forth in this chapter in mind as the book progresses and highlights the experiences of alienation, stigma, helplessness, pain, suffering, normlessness and turbulence which characterize the life course of terminally-ill hospital patients.

REFERENCES

1. A. Solzhenitsyn, *Cancer Ward*, Bantam Books, New York, 1969.
2. A. Gouldner, *The Dialectic of Technology and Ideology*, Seabury Press, New York, 1976.
3. U.S. Department of Health, Education and Welfare, Trends Affecting the United States Health Care System, DHEW publication no. HRA-7614503, January 1976.
4. E. Shils, Faith Utility and Legitimacy of Science, *Daedalus*, Summer, 1974.
5. B. Gendron, *Technology and the Human Condition*, St. Martin's Press, New York, 1977.
6. J. Ellul, *The Technological Society*, Vintage Books, New York, 1974.
7. N. Postman, *The Disappearance of Childhood*, Delacorte Press, New York, 1983.
8. J. Meyrowitz, *No Sense of Place: The Impact of Electronic Media on Social Behavior*, Oxford University Press, New York, 1985.
9. R. Nisbet, *The Quest for Community*, Oxford University Press, New York, 1981.
10. R. Bellah, et al., *Habits of the Heart*, University of California Press, Berkeley, 1985.
11. A. Etzioni, *An Immodest Agenda*, McGraw-Hill, New York, 1983.
12. P. Drucker, *Technology, Managment and Society*, Harper and Row, New York, 1970.
13. E. Fromm, *To Have Or To Be*, Bantam Books, New York, 1981.
14. J. Naisbitt, *Megatrends*, Warren Books, New York, 1984.
15. L. Tolstoy, *The Death of Ivan Ilych*, The New American Library, A Signet Book, New York, 1960.

CHAPTER
2

Death and Denial
in Modern America

... the idea of death, the fear of it, haunts the human animal like
nothing else; it is a mainspring of human activity—activity designed largely
to avoid the fatality of death, to overcome it by denying in some way that
it is the final destiny for man [1, p. ix].

Ernest Becker

Those who learned to KNOW death, rather than to fear and fight it, became our teachers about LIFE [2, p. xvii].

Elisabeth Kübler-Ross

In a society which seeks to conquer death through technology and does not have
firmly implanted systems of cultural support and meaning to legitimate and
make meaningful the experience of dying, it may be logical to expect the emergence of a widespread societal ethic of dying and death denial. In this chapter I
will discuss the idea of death denial from a sociological perspective, drawing
upon and furthering the themes of technology and self-expressiveness developed
in Chapter One.

In many ways, Americans conspire to keep death in a deep freeze of silent
avoidance. There is, if one surveys the social milieu of the contemporary American landscape, an obvious absence of death-related symbols, of conversation
geared toward dying and death, and an intriguing absence of popularized humor
about death and dying. This absence of death images and themes from ordinary
social intercourse bespeaks of a great silence about death, of what has been
termed in recent thanatology literature, the great cultural denial of death.

Death and the symbols of death have not always been absent from patterns
of everyday social living. In *The Hour of Our Death*, Ariès masterfully describes
how humanity traditionally defended itself against the threat of dying and death
through the use of ritual and community presence at the deathbed. Traditionally,
from the 5th up until the 19th century, an attitude of acceptance and unconcerned familiarity with death and its artifacts was socially widespread. The traditional patterns of human death reflected an intimacy of ongoing involvement
between human living and human dying. But as Ariès analyzes, the twentieth

century brought sweeping and radical changes to humanity's relation to death and dying. Dying, within the framework of the American 1980s and 1990s, has become stripped of religious and social significance and has, in some ways, become a sign of shame. Dying has, in the modern setting, been redefined into something dirty that takes place in social isolation and under the jurisdiction of medical and technological control. Ariès' description of the new world of death effectively illuminates how dying and death threaten the sensibilities of modern society:

> Death no longer inspires fear solely because of its absolute negativity; it also turns the stomach, like any nauseating spectacle. It becomes improper, like the biological acts of man, the secretions of the human body. It is indecent to let someone die in public. It is no longer acceptable for strangers to come into a room that smells of urine, sweat, and gangrene, and where the sheets are soiled. Access to this room must be forbidden, except to a few intimates capable of overcoming their disgust, or to those indispensable persons who provide certain services. A new image of death is forming: the ugly and hidden death, hidden because it is ugly and dirty [3, p. 569].

As dying and death become viewed as dirty, ways must be found to disinfect the processes of death. One major factor which facilitated the sanitizing of death was the transfer of death from the home and community to the hospital and the medical profession. Within the confines of the hospital or other medical facility, dying could be effectively circumscribed and controlled through technical, professional, and bureaucratic organization. In addition to the medicalization of death, dying has increasingly become a solitary experience. There is underlying truth to Woody Allen's comment that the difference between sex and death is that with death you do it alone and nobody laughs at you. As we saw in Chapter One, the process of dying is clearly affected by the deeply entrenched American value of individualism [4].

The organizing of modern death and dying within a medical-technical framework has precipitated the charge that American society is a death-denying society. Indeed, Glaser and Strauss have reported extensively on patterns of interaction between doctors, nurses, and patients, which deny, hide and obscure the realities of dying [5]. Sudnow, in an important study, discusses a variety of means by which death is literally and symbolically produced out of existence by the professional control of death in the hospital setting [6]. LeShan has found that, in seeking to avoid confronting the distasteful issue of dying, nurses construct a glass curtain, an impenetrable veil of silence between them and their patients. The function of this curtain of silence is to divert attention away from considerations of death [7]. Jay Katz, in his observations on patterns of doctor-patient communications, notes that doctors are very reluctant and unwilling to participate in the human, psychosocial issues that concern and shape the life-experiences of terminally-ill patients [8]. In a nutshell, these and other studies, have advanced the argument that the cultural framework of American society generates avoidance and denial of death and that the campaign for denial of and control over death is waged largely within the strictures of technological medicine.

On the other hand, there are a variety of factors present in American life today which seem to indicate that death is not denied as much as is claimed in the denial of death literature. Ironically, those scholars and others who have been writing about the American way of death denial over the past two decades or so, have been creating a body of academic and self-help type literature, the presence of which has served to undermine the societal denial of death. Some observers have gone as far as to comment that the recent attention given to death and dying has flooded the market with an overabundance of death-related discussion [9, pp. 1909-1910]. In addition, it has been argued that the theme of American death denial has been overstated. And, the fact that obituaries are printed daily in newspapers, hearses are regularly seen on public streets, sympathy cards are sold in ordinary stores, funeral parlors advertise in the Yellow Pages, etc., has been cited as an indicator that death is less than fully denied and hidden from the course of everyday affairs [10].

The idea of death-with-dignity has been brought to the attention of the general public through scholarly efforts, professional activities of health care personnel, the widespread social popularity of Elisabeth Kübler-Ross, and increasing media coverage of thanatology-related issues. The increased societal emphasis on the notion of death-with-dignity has also coincided with an increase in physician willingness to tell terminally-ill patients about their diagnosis. Traditionally, physicians have been reluctant to tell patients the truth about a terminal diagnosis for fear that the patient would "go to pieces" and become unmanageable upon hearing such news. Research during the fifties, sixties and early seventies indicated that physicians normatively believed that patients should not be told of a terminal condition, if non-disclosure was at all possible [11, pp. 86-94; 12, pp. 901-904; 13, pp. 11-21]. More recent studies, however, have shown that while there is not universal, professional agreement regarding what and how to tell a terminal patient of his or her diagnosis, physicians are increasingly coming to believe it is best to tell a patient with a terminal illness the truth and reassure them there is much that still can be done to treat them [14, pp. 57-63]. Although death attitudes of physicians are more conservative than attitudes of nurses, and doctors do typically still see death as a force to be conquered, physicians have become increasingly aware of the sociomedical issues relevant to the care of terminally-ill patients. Indeed, a majority of physicians have come to recognize that hospitals do have an obligation to meet the psychosocial needs of dying patients, and these same physicians also recognize that the needs of dying patients are being inadequately met by the present system of hospital care [15, pp. 333-334].

It would appear that the American relationship to death and dying is changing. The responses of seeking to avoid and deny seem to coexist alongside a recent societal thrust towards greater death openness. The unfolding of this relationship between the societal factors of "death avoidance" and "death acceptance" is bringing new understandings to the idea of death denial in American society. The key point to consider, however, is whether or not the thanatology movement, with its focus on death-with-dignity, represents a transformation of societal responses and attitudes to death or is consistent with the previously established framework of American death denial. Let us explore this issue of death and denial more fully.

The most challenging critique of the denial of death in human society is found in the scholarly thought of Ernest Becker. The starting point for Becker's analysis of death, society, and the human condition is the inherent vulnerability of the human species, especially in relationship to the certainty of death. Humanity, according to Becker, is born into an inescapable abyss of absurdity. He notes that by nature individuals are hopelessly absorbed with themselves (after all, luck is when the arrow hits the other guy), and in the spectrum of self-absorption there exists an insatiable craving to live; a craving which exists alongside of the knowledge that each of us must die. Becker argues that humanity is unable to accept what destiny has in store for us and that human life at this point becomes moved by the fear of death and the effort to transform the certainty of death into an illusion. As he opines, of all things that move humanity, one of the principal ones is the terror of death [1, p. 11]. Becker has the good sense to agree, however, with Jacques Choron's argument that it is impossible to determine concretely whether or not the fear of death is the core human anxiety. In this way, his entire body of thought on death denial stems from his association with a school of thought which sees death as the core motivational force of all societies. Even if the fear of death may seem to be absent in a given cultural context, Becker believes that the fear is being repressed, obscured and submerged by cultural forces. To his credit, Becker realizes he is stacking the deck. He can never intellectually lose his argument, as his response to factors which would seem to indicate humanity does not possess an overwhelming fear of death would be, "Oh, that's because they are repressing their fears." Not fair! Nevertheless, the framework of Becker's analysis does present a challenging case for the idea that culturally rooted behaviors and symbols represent an attempt to attain a sense of mastery over human mortality.

The fundamental intensity of humanity's fear of death has precipitated a natural human need to find ways to transcend death and deny mortality. It is this ubiquitous fear of death which drives the human species to seek transcendence of death through culturally shared hero systems and symbols [16, p. xvii]. Heroism is first and foremost the courage to stand up to death [1, p. 11]; it is the valiant individual who fearlessly looks death in the face. The hero has been the center of human admiration since the origin of civilization. When society honors a man or woman who bravely faces personal extinction, we acclaim the greatest victory humanity can achieve: triumph over death [1, p. 12]. Human society, with multiple ways and forms, continually seeks to secure victory over death; to offer to its citizens a sense of immunity from death.

Primitive societies extensively and heroically use rituals and ceremonies to shield their peoples from the evil of death and to furnish a set of explanations and meanings to mitigate the absurdities of life:

> Primitive man set up his society as a stage, surrounded himself with actors to play different roles, invented gods to address the performance to, and then ran off one ritual drama after the other, raising himself to the stars and bringing the stars down into the affairs of men. . . . And to think that when Western man first crashed uninvited into these spectacular dramas, he was scornful of what he saw. . . . Western man was being given a brief glimpse of the creations of human genius, and like a petulant imbecile bully who feels discomfort at what he doesn't understand, he proceeded to smash everything in sight [16, p. 15].

It was the ways of life and expressions of ritual which secured apotheosis for the vulnerable and technologically inept primitive. A triumph over death was accomplished through the myths, practices and symbols which allowed the living to enter the world of the dead and the dead to enter the world of the living. For this reason, primitive people were not as terrified of death as modern individuals. Their lives were usually secured and protected by a particular cultural ideology which in essence was an ideology of life and how to continue on and triumph over death [1, p. 45].

The observations of Ariès are also relevant at this point [3]. In his discussion of traditional and modern patterns of death and dying, he argues that going back to the 5th century, community presence, ritual, and everyday familiarity with death promoted an attitude of unconcerned acceptance of death and dying. In disagreeing with Becker, Ariès sees the traditional European ways of death as being essentially free from fear and denial. Many of the styles of living that shaped The Tame Death, The Death of the Self, Remote and Imminent Death, and the romanticized Death of the Other were so unabashedly open in their relationship to death and dying that it is difficult for modern individuals to grasp such societal patterns. Becker, in responding to Ariès, would argue that the eras of traditional death patterns were not free from denial nor fear, but rather gave rise to different forms of curtailing fear and denying death, than those which are so obvious in modern civilization. The interpretative differences of Ariès and Becker are interesting but the important point lies in their common recognition of the value of traditional patterns of ritual and ceremony in providing for comfort, solace, and even triumph in the haunting and inescapable shadow of death.

Ariès and Becker also agree that rituals to sustain the individual in the face of death have become empty, shallow and are even disappearing altogether. Ariès laments the absence of a societal response to death in modern society: society no longer observes a pause . . . everything . . . goes on as if nobody died anymore

[3, p. 560]. Becker, with broader intentions, argues that modern rituals have become hollow and unsatisfying, and as a result, modern society seeks to transcend death through science and greed. Becker points out that in the absence of stable and meaningful life rituals, human beings increasingly become "empty," "confused," and "impotent" during their lives and deaths [17, p. 24]. Men and women, therefore, increasingly seek to transcend their vulnerability and alienation through the pursuit of power, wealth, and any and all qualities that provide for the illusion of omnipotence and hence immortality. Becker takes his thesis to its logical conclusion and asserts that the fear of death and the need to deny this evil has been causally responsible for humanity bringing more evil into the world through power, greed and a heightening of destructive capacities.

Thus, for Becker, the stupidity of humanity lies in the nature of our social arrangements [17, p. 248]. Primitive peoples, up to a point, creatively designed rituals to deny death, rituals which enriched human experience. Modern society, in attempting to cope with the absence of meaningful rituals, has exploded onto a dangerous and irrational course of thirsting for power. The shallowness and instability of systems of explanation for life and death is creating a crisis of legitimacy for modern society. As a result, modern society seeks to deny death through promoting images of narcissism and invulnerability for everyday living, and through the heroic use of science and technology. Modern society is thus a hero system in that it stands up to death, helps the individual forget about death, and seeks to ultimately expunge death and dying from the framework of everyday social living.

Becker may be right in asserting that a consciousness of death is intolerable in a secular age, but his analysis fails to adequately establish the contention that the inability to "look at death in the face" must necessarily lead to denial. Indeed, to the contrary, the fear of death may be used as a catalyst for physicians to provide adequate and compassionate care to the needs of dying patients. In his discussion of death, fear, denial, and patient care, Momeyer begins by recognizing that denial of death ill suits one to give optimum care to dying patients. If the provider of care is denying and being motivated by his or her unacknowledged anxiety of death, a natural and logical result is the tendency to disinherit someone, namely the dying patient, whose circumstances are a source of anxiety [18, p. 8]. The literature reports how physicians' unwillingness to openly confront death often leads to neglect, over-treatment and insensitivity to the requirements of optimal patient care [19].[1] To the contrary, however, if health care providers honestly and openly acknowledge their fears of death, they enhance their ability

[1] For example, Fox's study of the professional socialization of medical students reveals how medical students are taught to submerge and hide their anxieties, fears and unease with the realities of death and dying. In this basic way, the system of medical training conspires to facilitate death denial among physicians and shackles their abilities to provide quality care to dying patients [19]. I will explore this in more detail in Chapter 3.

to maximally care for the dying patient. In this view, Momeyer argues that without recognition of one's own death-related fears, health professionals cannot offer the best care to their terminally-ill patients [19]. In relation to Becker's thesis, Momeyer's discussion instructs us that, on a personal level, fear of death does not have to lead to a 'psychologically adaptive attitude' of denial but can be used as a means of formulating strategies of patient care that are capable of transcending the restrictions of a denial-based pattern of care. One glaring omission of Becker's work, then, lies in his assumption that the 'inherent terror of death' must lead to denial. He never considers the possibility that humanity can find alternative ways to reconcile itself to the fearful certainty of human mortality.

Becker seeks to connect what he defines as escapist and capitalist behaviors with the collective human need to deny death. Consider, for example, an individual immersed in a crowd in a football stadium, his or her energies absorbed by the game, his or her loyalty to a team expressed through euphoria-promoting behaviors, all bound together by the excitement of winning. Becker interprets the widespread individual abandonment to the collective sports phenomenon in America as a means of escape, as a culturally promoted contrivance that helps the individual forget his or her vulnerabilities. In addition, Becker portrays the image of the insatiable pursuit of wealth and connects this obsession with the need to deny death, in that the accumulation of wealth lets one live on forever in the vicarious enjoyment of passing one's wealth to one's heirs [16, pp. 81-82]. Becker offers us captivating images and a compelling argument, but again he fails to establish causal linkages between the need for death denial and the scientific, capitalist and escapist pursuits of modern society. It is possible that an inverted relationship best characterizes death and societal response. One can logically advance the argument that our cultural preoccupation with materialism, narcissism, and technological progress has generated conditions of living, such as heightened individualism, decline in communal solidarity and increasing secularization, which are responsible for transforming dying and death into terrifying phenomena. Thus, those very factors which Becker identifies as responses to the terror of death may instead be etiological factors facilitating a fear of death:

> Becker's fateful assumption is that the fear of death leads to aggression and competition among people, and he never considers that the causal relationship may be the reverse, that the desperate death denying behavior he describes might be altered by a sense of connection and significance to other people that can be provided by genuinely communal relationships [20, p. 199].

There are, then, several factors which make Becker's thesis one dimensional and less than fully convincing. He sees death denial as being inherently initiated by the psychological human need to deny death and never considers that social structures can foster a dread of death or that social structures can be designed to diminish the fear of death and to even generate a societal ethos of accepting death. The failure to consider the historical scenarios portrayed by Illich, Ariès, Stannard and others leaves Becker's analysis interesting but incomplete. In addition, Becker's use of the concept of denial is so sweeping and all-encompassing that at times it becomes meaningless. Indeed, Becker, even by his own admission, uses the term "unfairly" to encompass every possible explanation for death-related behaviors. Similarly, in much of the thanatology literature there is a tendency to use the sweeping generalization of death denial in ways that are so encompassing and indiscriminately applied, that one has to wonder about the usefulness of the concept for explaining humanity's relation to death. In an intriguing review of the death-denial literature, Allan Kellehear argues that the term "denial" is too ill-defined, and its meaning is too broad for specific application and description [21, p. 717].

Kellehear also argues that it may be that modern society does not fear death so much as it fears dying. I commented in Chapter One that the way one dies is a reflection of the way one lives. Not only is this theme applicable to the lives of individuals, but also accurately accounts for the prevailing societal images of dying in a given time and place. In a culture where social support systems are low, individualism is emphasized, and technology is a prominent force, the idea of a cultural fear of death may be more correctly expressed as a fear of dying in isolation, indignity and meaninglessness. Death itself may not be as great a source of cultural terror as the dehumanization of human life during the process of dying. This denigration may be what human beings are finding most intolerable about death and dying in modern society (and this would be consistent with the implications of the human potential movement, discussed earlier). In this way, the most salient factor is not necessarily the fear of the cessation of life but of culture-spawned conditions of meaninglessness, stigma and suffering. Much of the patient experiences and commentary contained in the following chapters, supports the argument that the decimation of dignity and identity is the greatest source of fear and frustration for dying patients.

Dying is not so much denied in the sense that society ignores and makes the process of dying invisible, but rather dying is feared because of what it means for defilement, stigmatization and casting of dying people into the role of second-class citizens. Thus, on a societal level, the fear and denial of dying do not mean the complete avoidance of dying people and the facts of dying, but more correctly refer to the medicalization of life and death which has redefined the dying role into a low status, technology intensive, and potentially contaminating situation in need of sanitizing [21, p. 217].

The dying person constitutes a problem for the medical world in that he or she presents a *lingering*, often refractory, presence that is not immediately relievable by either cure or death.

We can learn much from the language used to describe the plight of dying people. Today, it has become commonly acceptable to use the work *lingering* in describing the life situation of a dying patient. Clearly, the idea of lingering was not an accurate reflector of the American way of dying fifty years ago, as the word itself would not have had much meaning within the social context of American society in the early part of the 20th century. I am reminded of the phrase *milk-run*, which was used to describe those missions of World War II pilots which were so regular and easily accomplished that the pilot could practically fly the mission with his eyes closed. The etymology of the phrase *milk-run* goes back to the days when milk was delivered to one's house in a horse-drawn cart. The milkman would journey the same delivery route in such a regular, stable, and predictable fashion that his horse would become able to travel the route, stopping where appropriate, without the explicit direction of the milkman. The idea of milk-run, with its textured pattern of regularity and stability, reflects a way of life that is rapidly vanishing from today's society. The idea of lingering, however, is a relevant descriptor of the modern way of dying in today's society. The widespread familiarity of the term *lingering* as a means of discoursing about dying, in and of itself, provides an insight into contemporary systems of living and dying. And the fact that the idea of lingering has become relevant at a time when the idea of milk-run is becoming irrelevant provides an additional commentary on the kinds of social forces that surround the modern experience of dying.

This point has been effectively illustrated in Leiderman and Grisso's study of "The Gomer Phenomenon." Gomers (*G*et *O*ut of *M*y *E*mergency *R*oom) epitomize the failure of technological medicine to eliminate illness and to heal the aging, as well as the failure of society to provide humane care for the socially isolated patient [22, p. 222]. Gomers, with their threatening presence of debilitating chronic illness, are sociomedically defined as low status patients. The seemingly inexorable decline which characterizes the career of Gomer patients, in their often confused and combative stages, underscores the impotence of modern, technological medicine. The image of a Gomer highlights the human fears of illness, intellectual decline, and loss of autonomy, as well as the doctor's frustration over the fact that modern medicine which promises to do much, too often fails to deliver on its promise [2, p. 231]. Like the Gomer, the dying person threatens to blemish the technological world of modern medicine.

It may be compelling to define societal and medical response to the problems presented by dying people in terms of death denial, but the idea of denial is useful only in a loose and approximate way. Physicians, dying patients, and family members may relate to death through the psychically rooted response of denial. However, when we speak on a societal and institutional level, death denial more precisely is a metaphor to describe a set of cultural, institutional, and structural responses to human dying and death. Kellehear thus concludes that societies do not deny death, but rather organize for it in ways that exert forms of social control through sanctioning different kinds of myths and rituals that determine culturally the nature of death, and set in motion processes of conflict, reintegration and adjustment of roles [21, p. 720]. In this process of organizing for death, modern society seeks to control, manage and contain the human processes of dying. The ways in which dying and death are managed and contained by the values, institutions and role expectations of a society are more sociologically useful in explaining humanity's relation to death and dying than the all-encompassing, snappy and descriptive term "denial" [23, pp. 285-290].

When we refocus our orientation from the idea of denial to the concept of *containing death and dying*, the seeming contradiction between America's orientation towards "death-denial" and the recent emphasis on death awareness can be readily reconciled.

The increased societal awareness of death and dying and the movement towards greater "acceptance" of death have been spawned by the work of Elisabeth Kübler-Ross. Not only has Kübler-Ross brought the issues of death and dying to the attention of the American public, she has been dubbed as a "secular saint" [24, p. 103] and a "charismatic religious leader" [25, pp. 89-109] by thanatology scholars as well as by her followers at Shanti Nilaya. Kübler-Ross has brought two recurrent messages to the attention of her followers and the general American public. The first of these, as indicated by the quotation that began this chapter, is that dying need not be something terrible and tragic but rather can be used as a springboard for courage, growth, enrichment, and joy. Her second and more recent message is even more ethereal and spiritual. Arguing that the affairs of this world are mundane and trivial, Kübler-Ross has steadfastly promoted the notion that physical life is merely a necessary prelude to "authentic experience," which she characterizes as the spiritual life of the self:

> You have to be in this temporary prison we call physical life, and you stay in this form until you have all of the positive experiences that this existence can afford you. But when you are in an energy pattern, you have access to all knowledge, understanding and unconditional love. You have all the wisdom of the universe [26, pp. 69-106].

The humanistic and spiritual messages of Kübler-Ross have had a great influence on the thanatology movement of the past two decades. The establishment of early hospices, the spread of death and dying courses on college campuses and increased media attention to the concept of death-with-dignity are, at least partially, a direct result of Kübler-Ross' articulation of the issues of death and dying. Her book, *On Death and Dying*, and the pictorial interview in the November 27, 1969 issue of *Life* magazine catapulted Kübler-Ross into fame and public attention. Personal appearances on television, growing attention in local and national newspapers and magazines, coupled with her outstanding skills as a communicator quickly established Kübler-Ross as the leading authority on care of the dying. Although she was involved only minimally with the hands-on-care of dying patients or in the implementation of hospice programs in America, Kübler-Ross has become synonymous with death and dying in American society.

She has become the dominant spokesperson for the needs of dying patients, the idea of death-with-dignity, and the hospice movement.

As we saw in Chapter One, American culture was and is ready for "Kübler-Ross' Thanatology Movement." In our era of individualism, the concept of death as a final stage of growth is consistent with the value of self-actualization. The human potential movement, then, with its orientation toward therapeutic intervention and amelioration, has set the stage for the spread of clinical/psychological management of the dying. It is in this way that the hospice, while being a structural outgrowth of the death-awareness movement, is also logically reflective of the underlying American value of individualism and self-actualization.

The major mission of the hospice is to assist patients and families to meet the burdens and challenges of dying with as much creativity and dignity as possible [27, p. 207]. The idea of death-with-dignity, while talked about quite a bit, however, is elusive to define. As one surveys the everyday operational realities of the hospice, it becomes apparent that the control of discomfort has become the major focus of the hospice program of caring for the terminally-ill. In their "little recipe-book" on the management of terminal disease, Cicely Saunders and Mary Baines offer, from a social-clinical perspective, a snapshot of the issues involved with the care of dying patients, with particular emphasis on the management of pain. Relevant sections of their book are entitled "use of analgesics for terminal pain," "adjuvant therapies for pain control," and "control of symptoms other than pain" [28]. In the situation where cure or life prolongation are no longer viable options, the hospice seeks to manage the dying process through the amelioration of symptoms. When pain and other symptoms are controlled or minimized, multidisciplinary hospice teams can then turn their attention to the myriad psychological, social and spiritual concerns of the patient and his or her family [29, p. 19].

As one surveys the hospice literature, the themes of comfort, pain management, and enhancement of the living process are repeated over and over again. It is not pushing too far to suggest that the ultimate management and treatment objective of hospice care is the "normalization" of life; the facilitation and sustenance of ordinary, everyday styles of living (or as close as possible thereto). It is in this way that the hospice and death-with-dignity movement can be seen, within the framework articulated by Becker, as hero systems over death. In the hospice framework of living, the extraordinary and the horrible have become reduced to the ordinary and the "natural." Sounds of discontent and the howls of anguish are channeled into silent whispers of acceptance. Indeed, the hospice by its thrust to defeat the anxieties and fears of death becomes a philosophy and structure that achieves a triumph over death. Through its emphasis on living fully and maximizing life in death's shadow, along with its deep connections to religion, the hospice secures for the dying patient a victory over his or her limitations and vulnerabilities.

The essential point to emphasize is that the point of merger for strategies designed to avoid or 'deny' death, the aggressive technical management of the dying, and the entire death-with-dignity movement, is that each of these responses to death represents a form of trying to control or to contain the human course of death and dying. It is my contention that as society organized to contain death through rituals and other forms of cultural legitimation during the ages of traditional death patterns, modern society seeks to contain the potentially disruptive consequences of human dying through the rituals and philosophy of the death-with-dignity movement and through the technological control and management of the human dying problem.

Thus, while there appears to be no single direction to the thanatology literature, we have seen how varying and apparently contradictory forces converge to provide a societal and medical program for the control, management and containment of human death. The remainder of this book will be concerned with how the values of technocratic society are reflected in the care of dying patients in the hospital setting and how the hero system of technocratic consciousness and medical-technical management of the dying shape the course of the terminal life experience.

REFERENCES

1. E. Becker, *The Denial of Death*, The Free Press, New York, 1973.
2. E. Kübler-Ross, *On Children and Death*, Collier Books, New York, 1983.
3. P. Ariès, *The Hour of Our Death*, Alfred Knopf, New York, 1981.
4. D. Stannard, *The Puritan Way of Death*, Oxford University Press, New York, 1976.
5. B. Glaser and A. Strauss, *Awareness of Dying*, Aldine, New York, 1965.
6. D. Sudnow, *Passing On*, Prentice-Hall, New Jersey, 1967.
7. L. LeShan, Psychotherapy and the Dying Patient, in *Death and Dying*, L. Pearson (ed.), Case Western Reserve University Press, Cleveland, 1969.
8. J. Katz, *The Silent World of Doctor and Patient*, The Free Press, New York, 1984.
9. S. Vasirub, Dying Is Worked to Death, *The Journal of the American Medical Association, 229*:14, September 30, 1980.
10. R. Kalish, *Death, Grief and Caring Relationships*, Brooks/Cole, California, 1985.
11. D. Oken, What to Tell Cancer Patients, *The Journal of the American Medical Association, 175*, pp. 86–94, 1961.
12. W. T. Fitts and I. S. Ravin, What Philadelphia Physicians Tell Patients with Cancer, *The Journal of the American Medical Association, 153*, pp. 901–904, 1953.
13. R. Schulz and D. Aderman, How the Medical Staff Copes with Dying Patients, *Omega 7*:11, pp. 11–21, 1976.
14. C. B. Hatfield et al., Attitudes about Death, Dying and Terminal Care: Differences among Groups at a University Teaching Hospital, *Omega, 14*:1, 1983.
15. J. E. Kincade, Attitudes of Physicians, Housestaff and Nurses on Care for the Terminally Ill, *Omega, 13*:4, 1983.

16. E. Becker, *Escape from Evil*, The Free Press, New York, 1975.
17. ⸻, *The Structure of Evil*, The Free Press, New York, 1968.
18. R. Momeyer, Fearing Death and Caring for the Dying, *Omega, 16*:1, 1985.
19. R. Fox, The Autopsy: Attitude Learning of Second Year Medical Students, in *Essays in Medical Sociology*, John Wiley and Sons, New York, 1979.
20. A. Killilea, Death and Social Consequences, *Omega, 11*:3, 1980.
21. A. Kellehear, Are We a Death Denying Society? A Sociological Review, *Social Science and Medicine, 18*:9, 1984.
22. D. Leiderman and J. A. Grisso, The Gomer Phenomenon, *Journal of Health and Social Behavior, 25*, p. 222, September 1985.
23. P. Donaldson, Denying Death: A Note Regarding Some Ambiguities in the Current Discussion, *Omega, 3*:3, 1972.
24. L. Lofland, *The Craft of Dying*, Sage Publications, Beverly Hills, 1978.
25. D. Klass and R. Hutch, Elisabeth Kübler-Ross as a Religious Leader, *Omega 16*:2, 1985–86.
26. Playboy Interview: Elisabeth Kübler-Ross, *Playboy, 28*:5, 1981.
27. T. Gonda and J. E. Ruark, *Dying Dignified: The Health Professional's Guide to Care*, Addison-Wesley, California, 1984.
28. C. Saunders and M. Baines, *Living With Dying: The Management of Terminal Disease*, Oxford University Press, Oxford, 1983.
29. I. Ajemian and B. Mount, The Adult Patient: Cultural Considerations in Palliative Care, in *Hospice: The Living Idea*, Cicely Saunders (ed.), W. B. Saunders Co., Philadelphia, 1981.

CHAPTER 3

Technological Medicine, the Technocratic Physician and Human Dying

Doctor, just don't do something, stand there!

Oliver Wendell Holmes

Death is not the enemy, Doctor. Inhumanity is.

Male Patient

I almost had a croaker upstairs!

W. L. J., M.D.

The technological base of American medicine is a reflection of the techno-logical underpinnings of the broader social order. Constant efforts at discovery exerted by the scientific community, the industrial and public fascination with technological developments and the important place these developments play in shaping medical progress are evidence of society's general willingness to accept and place faith in the technocratic ethos. It is for these reasons that the structure and orientation of the everyday, technical activities of the medical profession is a logical extension of the technological foundation of society. The purpose of this chapter is to evaluate technological medicine as a means of managing the dying patient, keeping in mind my previous discussion of technocracy, and underscoring the role of technology in shaping the doctor-patient relationship.

A physician's training is a major determinant of the manner in which he or she will relate to patients in general and dying people in particular. Medical students generally face their first sustained encounter with death in the anatomy lab during their first year of study. The experience, for a young twenty-two or twenty-three-year-old, of anticipating and walking into the anatomy laboratory, with an array of cadavers awaiting attention, inevitably and profoundly affects the students and their perceptions of patient care. Indeed, the anatomy lab experience is a watershed in the socialization process of student doctors.

A cadaver, cool to the touch, breathless, mummified, of macabre substance and of sickly pallor, initially is a source of anxiety for the medical student.

Meeting one's cadaver is a memorable and emotionally significant experience, and often becomes a focus of intense emotional activity for the medical student. Naming the cadaver, joking about it in a way that has been commonly described as gallows-humor, and repressing any outward sign of anxiety or discomfort in deference to maintaining a nonchalant attitude, are standard responses of the medical student to the anatomy lab experience. As one student comments:

> My cadaver's name is Helen. She's really kind of gross . . . had a breast removed. . . . You deal with them very casually. Like eventually one part of her anatomy was removed and placed up another part, if you know what I mean . . .

Another student adds:

> I just couldn't believe that everybody else was as unaffected as they appeared. I had never been more terrified in my life.

The tumultuous emotional response to the cadaver and its being studied, explored, and dissected is quickly smoothed over and replaced by an attitude of emotional disinterest and detachment. Thus, as we can see from the above comments, by restraining and containing their emotional responses, students swiftly learn to isolate their attention on technical and scientific considerations. In addition to gathering knowledge that is important to development as a student physician, the student begins to learn something more subtly expressed but yet essential to the present definition of medical care of patients. He or she is socialized by the anatomy experience, and its role-behavioral expectations, into an objective, emotionally neutral, and technologically oriented world view. In important ways, the medical student learns a pattern of relating to future patients through the patterns by which he or she relates to the cadaver. In some ways the cadaver is an ideal patient. In addition to being a haven for technical and physical exploration, it is emotionally undemanding, passively acquiescent, and fully cooperative. These are qualities, of course, inherent to a cadaver, which the medical student comes to value as appropriate behavioral expectations for future (living) patients.

The observations of Renée Fox in her eloquent essay on the autopsy and socialization of second-year medical students are also relevant here. Fox observes that like the anatomy lab experience, in addition to imparting important medical knowledge and skills, the autopsy serves to transmit attitudes and values which are salient to the prevailing definition of a physician's role. More specifically, by providing students with a real workout in objectivity, the experience fertilizes the seeds of emotional detachment that are planted the year before in anatomy lab. This way, as Fox notes, the most potent impact of the autopsy is in the realm of training students for detached concern [1, 56].

Fox begins her account by contrasting the cadaver experience with the psychosocial impact of the autopsy. She observes that the autopsy has a greater link with human life than the cadaver confronted in the anatomy lab. The body is

often still warm, is not mummified, will bleed when cut into, and is legally protected by concern for the family and impending funeral. This awareness of the
human dimensions of the deceased, is articulated by a second year student:

> When you see the initial incision and first bleeding, that's a point at
> which you are very aware of the whole person. . . . You realize that this
> is someone who has died, and that what you are going to do is look inside
> that person . . . [1, p. 58].

Fox makes the point that, because of its greater connection to human life,
the autopsy poses greater emotional difficulty for the medical student. While effectively pointing to the greater resemblance to human life of the corpse to be
autopsied, Fox, however, tends to minimize the significance of a student's very
first professional encounter with the dissection of a dead human body. It may be
methodologically difficult to accomplish, but the role of the first (cadaver) experience in preparing the student for the second (autopsy) experience needs to
be studied with particular attention being paid to whether the experience in the
anatomy lab and first year of study in general helps to desensitize students to
the emotional trauma posed by one's initial autopsy experience. Clearly, the
seeds of emotional detachment are sown in the first year of study and, as Fox's
work indicates, the growth of the qualities of detachment and objectivity are
nurtured by the autopsy experience. In this sense, Fox's distinction artificially
fragments what needs to be seen as a continuous and comprehensive program of
professional socialization throughout the entirety of a medical student's years
of study.

The role that the autopsy plays in shaping the technocratic consciousness of
detachment, objectivity, and rationality, however, is most effectively described
by Fox. The autopsy, with the social role expectations of both teachers and
students, demands that exclusive attention be given to the facts of the case, to
become so "engrossed in the scientific angles that the emotional aspects are obscured:"

> Now when I see a lung, for example, I concentrate on its structure . . .
> I don't picture its being someone who was once living, breathing, and talk-
> ing. . . . [1, p. 63].
> Most of the fellows are so eager to be good doctors that they force
> themselves to look at things in a scientific way. . . . Every guy was inter-
> ested in the facts . . . asking questions and wanting to learn about what
> had happened [1, p. 63].

In short, the autopsy facilitates the emergence of an attitude of depersonal-
ized regard of the corpse being autopsied in particular and towards the phenomenon of death in general. Since the focus of the watershed experiences of the
anatomy lab and the autopsy is technical, as is the thrust of all years of medical
training and socialization, young medical students are taught about the centrality
of technical activity in relating to patients and to death. And, as we shall now

see, despite variations in form, the common underlying dimension which characterizes the manner in which physicians relate to dying patients is the technical world view.

The collective medical approach to the care of dying patients is eminently technological. Despite the fact that there is increasing variation in the styles and behaviors which characterize the interrelationships between doctors and their patients, there is a strong behavioral and attitudinal commonality in the way physicians normally relate to each other in the backstage arenas of medicine with regard to the care of terminally-ill patients. I have observed that the private discussions of formal inter-physician consultations and informal conversations about the condition of dying patients tend to be decidedly detached and sometimes quite callous. In the absence of a patient's physical presence, physicians are personally and professionally free to relate to the process of a patient's dying in ways which are similar to the nature of their relationship to the cadaver in the anatomy lab. Thus, in many ways, backroom joking about patients, defilement of physical or social selves of patients, and objectifying the human plight of their circumstances, casts the care of dying patients into the detached realm of "cadaver-treatment." Consider the following hallway conversation between a surgeon and an oncologist regarding what they should tell a patient whose leg biopsy had just come back positive and whose chest x-rays had revealed progression of an already identified tumor:

Surgeon:	This is a bad, aggressive disease. We are talking months.
Oncologist:	He really can't be irradiated to his chest. His Adriamycin isn't working. He's on full dosage, and his disease is progressing.
Surgeon:	But we have to do something for him.[1]
	PAUSE . . .
Surgeon:	I'm not impressed with his moral fiber. I don't think he has the moral strength to withstand the news. His family also impresses me as being weak. I don't think they have the strength to cope with the consequences of someone dying . . . So, what do we tell him?
Oncologist:	Well, we have to tell him that his biopsy was positive, but we also need to assure him that we are not going to give up on him.
Surgeon:	Yes, but you really can't irradiate his chest. He's going to drown from his disease, and you don't want to make it worse for him by his catching radiation fibrosis and drowning from that.
Oncologist:	Then that'll help his drowning . . .
Surgeon:	Okay. We'll tell him that the femur biopsy was positive and that we want to treat it with x-rays.
Oncologist:	What about the lung? We have to tell him something.

[1]In and of itself, this is a powerful statement about the heroism of the technological management and manipulation of death.

Surgeon:	We'll tell him that we are watching some areas closely . . . that some areas seem to be suspicious.

This backstage-hallway conversation enabled the physicians to develop a protective strategy that would guide them through the tasteless task of delivering bad news to the patient. It is interesting, especially in light of the newly inspired emphasis on truth telling within medical circles, that the physicians decided to tell the patient the truth—nothing but the truth—but not the whole truth. And, as we shall see in greater detail in Chapter Seven, focusing attention and energy on specific symptoms is a useful means of diverting attention away from the harsh and truthful realities of dying to the *more manageable concern of symptom treatment*. In this way, truth is told but truths about dying are averted. It is precisely this process of "partial truth telling" which enables physicians to salve their consciences in light of the movement toward open awareness of dying and the patient's right to know, while simultaneously protecting themselves from having to deal directly with the issue of dying.

This fancy footwork around the truth-of-the-truth is rooted in the patient's best interest, as explained by the medical profession. The patient has enough to worry about, it is argued, without being confronted with harsh and naked, truthful realities which may destroy all semblance of hope. And, as we witnessed in the above scenario, it is often believed that the unveiling of the whole truth will irretrievably shatter the lives of patients and their families. In reality, however, the avoidance of full disclosure, avoidance of telling the basic truth and all of its implications, can deleteriously affect the lives of patients and serve ultimately the interests of doctors.

Let us now return to the hospital floor and listen in on how the patient was actually told "the truth."

The surgeon proceeds from the hallway to the patient's room while the oncologist temporarily goes down to the doctors' lounge to take care of some business. The surgeon enters the room and sits in a chair to the right of the patient's bed with the tray stand between him and the patient. After a brief exchange of pleasantries, the surgeon begins:

Surgeon:	We got the results of the biopsy back, and there was a tumor in it.
Patient:	There was?!
Surgeon:	Yes.
Patient:	But, I thought you said you had gotten it out.
Surgeon:	Yes, but I also said there was a possibility that it may come back. That is why we want to treat it with x-rays. PAUSE . . .
Patient:	How effective is the x-rays? . . . Does it work? . . . Will it work for me? What are my chances?
Surgeon:	I really can't say. It varies tremendously. 100 percent from individual to individual. I can't tell you what your chances are. Those who succeed do so 100 percent; those who fail are 100

	percent failures. It makes no sense for me to quote you sta-
	tistics. Either you as an individual will succeed or not.
Patient:	So, therefore, if we succeed, my chances are 100 percent, and
	if not, then we are somewhere in the middle.
	PAUSE ... NO RESPONSE FROM THE SURGEON
Patient:	Is the leg the only biopsy which you did?
Surgeon:	Yes, only on the leg.
Patient:	Then I only have cancer in my leg?
Surgeon:	Well, ... [PAUSE] ... We did take some x-rays, and we do
	want to watch your chest closely.
	[ONCOLOGIST COMES IN AND SITS ON THE BEDSIDE]
Patient:	What did the x-rays show?
Surgeon:	There's some areas that seem to be suspicious, and we want to
	watch them very closely.
Patient:	Will you treat those areas with x-rays?
Surgeon:	No, but that's Dr. _____'s department. [nods to the on-
	cologist].
Oncologist:	We want to get you started on radiation for your leg as soon
	as possible, and we'll be watching to see if chemotherapy is
	indicated. If we do opt for chemotherapy, it will be of a mild-
	er form than the combination you are now on with Adria-
	mycin.
Patient:	Will you still continue to give me that?
Oncologist:	No.
Patient:	When will I be getting radiation?
Oncologist:	Well, we have to talk to you about that. About where you are
	going to get treated, here or at home.
	[CONVERSATION TURNS TO A DISCUSSION OF THE
	CONVENIENCE OF THE PATIENT'S LOCAL HOSPITAL
	VS. THE MEDICAL CENTER WHERE HE WAS PRESENT-
	LY ADMITTED]
	... PAUSE ...
Surgeon:	Anything else? ... Do you have any questions for us?
Patient:	No, it's just that I didn't expect things to go bad so quickly.
	[in deep and somber reflection]
Oncologist:	Yes, but you have been informed that cancer is an aggressive
	disease that can spread like wildfire—very rapidly. That's why
	we want to watch you closely and give you the very latest and
	best treatment available.
	[FLOW OF CONVERSATION STYMIED] ... PAUSE ...
Surgeon:	[getting up to leave] Mr. ———————, if you have any other
	questions, feel free to ask us. We're around, write them down
	so you don't forget.

The irony of the foregoing doctor-patient interaction is that it accomplished precisely the opposite of what the surgeon intended in his hallway discussion. The patient by his own words ("I just didn't expect things to go bad so quick-ly") realizes that his condition is critically serious, despite all of the elaborate jugglery of the surgeon and even the oncologist in spots. But, in many ways the central issue revolves around clarity and ambiguity in the process of truth telling.

In other words, it is an issue of the various meanings that can be associated with and emerge from the telling of truth. Physicians, by nature of their role definition, have a comprehensive picture of the patient's diagnosis and prognosis, but the various strategies employed by doctors in telling a patient of his or her diagnosis often provide for the patient a correct but murky understanding of their own life-disease situation. In this way, a haunting "shadow of awareness" surrounds the patient. The understanding of his or her circumstances is often accompanied with, as one patient put it, "anxiety about what they are not telling me." In addition, a further irony is introduced into the framework of patient care, namely, that patients who are defined as too weak or "morally inferior" to face up to the whole truth are presumed to have sufficient moral fiber and personal strength to wade through the ambiguities associated with partial truth telling and to cope with the ragings of their own imaginations. It is clear from the materials we have just considered that, while physicians may believe they are protecting their patients by disguising the telling of truth, their dancing around the truth-of-the-truth largely reflects their own unease in dealing directly with dying and its tribulations. If it really is in the best interest of patients to protect them from the whole truth, then patients should be wholly protected. The patient should be told nothing and even lied to if necessary.

Present day realities of truth telling are influenced by increasing pressures from the death-with-dignity movement and the doctor's own and changing awareness of the dimensions of this movement. Another relevant factor is inadequate professional training and socialization of doctors in the area of the psychosocial care of patients and, in particular, dying patients. In this way, contemporary physicians find themselves embodied in a situation of ambiguity, of feeling the societal pressures towards open death awareness but not having been trained to feel at ease with the open-awareness framework. For this reason, there is an absence of sociomedically sanctioned norms to guide physicians in truth-telling behaviors. Physicians as a result are left to their own resources in devising strategies to tell their patients bad news.

As discussed earlier, technology is the main coordinating force of the medical profession and of medical training. However, this does not mean to imply that physicians relate to their patients in a monolithic, unvarying way. As there are differences in the ways physicians approach truth telling, there are a variety of patterned ways by which physicians relate to dying patients. These ways are not fixed nor invariable throughout the career of a physician. In the absence of standardized norms that define how doctors should relate to patients, it is possible for physicians to oscillate among various patterns and to treat one patient differently from another.

One major patterned response of the physician to the process of dying is direct and active technical intervention. This orientation, whereby the physician strives officiously to keep his or her patients alive, has been extensively discussed in the literature. I have found that interns and residents are especially eager to employ and "over-employ" the skills of their profession, to "save at all costs" a patient with a rapidly progressing terminal condition. Younger physicians are understandably proud and enthusiastic about their achievements, and it is not difficult to see how the technical powers they have amassed can lead them toward a developing sense of omniscience. It becomes difficult for many physicians, in light of the societal and medical value of technological activism, the devaluation of dying and the professional socialization of doctors, to simply "stand there and do nothing." Such passivity in the face of death is inconsistent with the flow of modern values and against the grain of physicians' consciousness. Hence, when physicians, and this is especially relevant for young "unexperienced" doctors, are confronted with the realities of human suffering and dying, they will resort to what they are most familiar with to help them cope with the threats of dying, namely, technical intervention and activity.

Throughout much of the popularized and academic thanatology literature, the save-at-all-costs orientation is associated with the heroics of transplants, connecting patients to life-prolonging machines, miracles of surgery and other technological triumphs. However, the daily unfolding of the save-at-all-costs orientation of the profession is not so dramatic as the medical headlines which capture the attention of society at large. Rather, everyday medical practice is best characterized by the regular, ongoing belief that the doctor's job is to promote and prolong life through technically aggressive patterns of care. In this way, the save-at-all-costs orientation is ubiquitous in the profession. Variations occur when some doctors supplement their care of patients with practices that go beyond technical considerations. Other doctors recognize that one can reach a costly and useless point of no return on technical activity for dying patients. These physicians frequently proceed to direct their energies elsewhere rather than spend them aggressively seeking a technical cure of the dying patient.

A second orientation to the care of the dying is avoidance-neglect. A patient who is dying and not responding to treatment can become a difficult patient for some doctors. Those physicians who define their role exclusively in terms of curing (as opposed to caring) will naturally tend to spend their time and energy in the treatment of those patients, seriously ill or otherwise, who have a reasonable chance of responding to the doctor's curative therapies.

It needs to be stressed that doctors do not generally make a conscious decision to neglect their patients. Neglect is frequently an unintentional consequence of the doctor's unease in dealing with terminal patients, coupled with a commitment to other patients that are defined as a primary priority. One patient tells the story of how she was informed that she had developed cancer in her breast:

> I was in the clinic after being examined, waiting for the doctor to return with my test results. He came in and told me to get dressed. Even when he said, "I have to talk to you," I was not worried.
> Then he came out and told me I had breast cancer. He was abrupt, real abrupt. He had other patients to see, and he went off to see them.

I don't know how I made it. I walked out in tears . . . alone. . . . I was alone for over half an hour, wandering around the hospital. There was no hospital or medical support. The doctor left me, and I found myself facing this myself.

Stories like this abound as patients recount their experiences with the medical profession. Some scenarios are dramatic in terms of neglect,[2] others less so, but the common denominator of the spectrum of avoidance-neglect behaviors is the unwillingness of the physician to give of the time it takes to adequately care for the needs of dying patients.

From the doctor's perspective, what may appear as neglect is really medical prioritizing. As one physician comments:

Yes, it's true that some of these patients receive less care than others. But there are only so many hours in the day, and decisions have to be made on who are going to receive the most beneficial results from our attention. For example, today I've had. . . .

Sudnow's study, almost twenty years ago, pointed to the same phenomenon: physicians' defining their role in terms of activity that would medically benefit patients [2]. It is fascinating to note how much remains the same in terms of the prioritizing of physician activity in the realm of technical activity and how this obsession with technologically-based amelioration of disease jeopardizes the plight of dying patients. Indeed, as Anselm Strauss puts it, "I too am amazed at how little the technological base of hospital care has changed over the past twenty-five years."[3]

A third pattern of care of the dying is detached-sympathetic-support. There are physicians, and the thanatology movement is instrumental here, who believe that the physical-technical care of dying patients needs to be complemented with psychosocial considerations. The sympathetically oriented physician recognizes and freely speaks of the need for social and psychological support systems in the care of the dying. The detached-sympathetic-support physician is generally aware of how often the medical and hospital structure of patient care minimizes the importance of these considerations. However, this type of physician most frequently does not direct activities toward changing these structural realities, but rather is satisfied with his or her own awareness of the emotional and social needs of the dying.

Also, it is important to note that detached-sympathetic-support physicians are typically reluctant to indict other physicians, including interns and residents,

---

[2] I have observed doctors leaving patients stranded in hospital beds awaiting various procedures while the doctors have been out of town or otherwise unavailable, doctors refusing to continue seeing particular patients, doctors making every effort to see patients when they were asleep or scheduled for tests so they wouldn't have to interact with patients, as well as doctors paying such minimal attention to the case of a patient that the patient's health was jeopardized.

[3] Personal communique regarding his review/evaluation of an earlier form of this book.

for attending inadequately to the psychosocial needs of dying patients. This is not true in the medical or technical arena, however. When medically or technically relevant mistakes or abuses occur, these mistakes often elicit responses from physicians, who are correctly seeking to protect the best interests of their patients. If mistakes are made by housestaff doctors, strong corrective sanctioning is frequently used. If abuses or mistakes result from the activity of established colleagues, more informal, softer methods of addressing the issue are generally employed. In any event, medically relevant neglect, abuse or mistakes are an explicit issue of concern for the professional world view of physicians. This means that concern over the technical competence of patient care is formally built into the professional milieu of physicians. Concern for the psychosocial dimensions of patient care is not a structural, institutionalized part of the organization of contemporary medical practice. It exists to the degree that physicians, especially detached-sympathetic-support physicians, make private, individualized statements about the value of psychosocial factors of patient care. This statement typically is made through specific and individualized patterns of care and is not formally part of an expressed doctrine or ideology of care. In this way, attention to the psychosocial needs of dying patients is not an established pattern of physician behavior. Rather, it exists on an individualized level of expression, that is to say, it becomes a personal and individualized folkway of patient care.

It is important to recognize that the detached-sympathetic-support physician has not been socialized in a different manner from other medical colleagues, but rather makes an individual statement about his or her definition of appropriate patterns of patient care. This way of responding to the needs of dying patients is generally not informed by formal psychosocial training (most physicians never even take a course in death and dying), but rather represents a personal, informal, and self-expressive effort to bring a sense of compassion to the practice of medicine. In this way, the physician's approach to the care of patients is consistent with the values of individualism and self-expression, already discussed. In addition, despite the fact that more physicians are becoming aware of the need for psychosocial care of the dying, sympathetic-support physicians are still mavericks in that there is little formal, structural sanctioning and support of their non-technical activities.

The primary difference I have observed between detached-sympathetic-support physicians and others lies in their willingness to listen to patient complaints, to spend more time in formal professional interaction with patients, and to participate in informal conversation with patients. I have witnessed patterns of behavior that include touching patients in nontechnical situations (reassuring hand on the arm, shoulder, etc.), consistently and explicitly responding to the comfort needs of patients and to the dignity needs of patients, e.g. privacy, bodily integrity, etc. It is these qualities of patient care which provide a commitment to a broader spectrum of care than that formally taught in medical school and formally sanctioned by peer review and approval.

However, the central and primary focus of the detached-sympathetic-support physician is technically based. The primary goal still is disease and symptom treatment and the technological amelioration of pain and discomfort. Thus, the care that is provided by the sympathetic physician is similar to that of the save-at-all-costs and avoidance-neglect physician. It is the forms of care that appear to be quite different. Some unrelentingly pursue the cure of their patients, others prioritize their technical efforts towards treating more medically-responsive patients, and the detached-sympathetic-support physician seeks to provide the best technical care possible in a way that is tempered by humane and psycho-social considerations. The underlying factor of these varying forms of patient care is a technological focus and technological activity, the function of which is to manage, control, and contain the process of dying through the doctor's personalized and varying application of the technological ethos.

When a patient nears the threshold of death, some doctors seek to avoid death through heroics, others avoid death by turning their attention elsewhere, and others seek to make the patient as comfortable as possible. However, despite the necessity of interacting in varying degrees with dying patients when death is near, physicians uniformly strain to move psychically and physically away from the death setting, as quickly as they can. I have noticed a formal and regular rush to move on to the next patient and on to another floor, when doctors are cast into a situation where death is imminent. Additionally, discussion of the dying patient during the final phase of life becomes increasingly euphemistic, detached, and technically narrow. Consider the following round-robin discussion in the doctors' lounge of a patient with a fourteen-year history of myeloma, who was approaching her death and was lingering at the threshold thereof:

Intern:	This could be it.
Oncologist 1:	I don't know what the future holds for her. PAUSE . . .
Neurologist:	Well, my husband is cooking a roast beef tonight. I'm going home and have dinner . . .
Intern:	[speaking to Oncologist 1] What do you think, is Mrs._____ going to have some platelets for dinner?
Oncologist 1:	[concerned and in brief but deep thought] I don't know what to do for her.
Intern:	Well, do you want to say good-bye to her tonight?
Oncologist 1:	She's on autopilot now. Either she makes it or she doesn't. Let's leave her alone.
Intern:	Okay.
Oncologist 2:	[speaking to Oncologist 1] I think it's time for _____ to leave us. The pity of the whole thing though, is that we will not get an autopsy.
Oncologist 1:	Oh, that's something I'm going to insist on!

In summary, with the exception of the technological foundation of physician activity, there is increasing normlessness with respect to the definition of how physicians should relate to dying patients. The recent thanatology movement with its emphasis on death awareness and death-with-dignity has conflicted with the traditional medical approach of not telling terminally-ill patients about their diagnosis. As a result, the men and women of medicine are embarking on a personal and group search to decide how much and in what fashion to tell their patients. Additionally, there are no firmly established behavioral patterns to direct the physician during the course of interactions with the dying. The irony of this situation is that as medical technology is becoming more rational, calculable, and definitive, the more uncertainty and confusion are being introduced into interactions between physicians and dying patients.

The professional socialization of doctors is woefully inadequate in providing a satisfactory base of training to assist physicians in establishing stable and effective patterns of interaction with dying patients. The inadequacy of their professional training makes patterns of interacting with dying patients something that physicians must carve out individually. It is understandable within this framework of inadequate education, normlessness, and confusion on the part of physicians themselves, that personal and professional ambiguity will oftentimes result in inconsistent behavior, abrupt bedside manner, and even abuse and neglect.

Physicians are, however, bonded together through their commitment to technological activity. Clearly, technology is the driving force in medical education. Clearly, technological activism is the dominant factor which shapes the world view of physicians. Clearly, the technological orientation of the medical profession is the major force which shapes physician interaction with dying patients. Thus, despite the realities of normlessness and the appearance of differences in the approach of doctors to the treatment of the dying patient, technology is the pre-eminent tool used in the management of the terminally-ill.

It is interesting to observe that after all the attention to death-related issues engineered by Kübler-Ross and the death-with-dignity proponents, little has changed in the core values, structure, and orientation of the medical management of dying patients.

REFERENCES

1. R. Fox, The Autopsy: Attitude Learning of Second Year Medical Students, in *Essays in Medical Sociology*, John Wiley and Sons, New York, 1979.
2. D. Sudnow, *Passing On*, Prentice Hall, Englewood Cliffs, New Jersey, 1967.

CHAPTER
4

Individualism, Fellowship and Dying

Think of what it must be for a dying man, trapped behind hundreds of walls . . . , while the whole population, sitting in cafés or hanging on the telephone, is discussing shipments, bills of lading, discounts! It will then be obvious what discomfort attends death, even modern death, when it waylays you under such conditions [1, p. 5].[1]

Albert Camus

She died a week later. When Garp went to her room, it was whisked clean, the bed stripped back, the windows wide open. When he asked for her, there was a nurse in charge of the floor whom he didn't recognize—an iron-gray maiden who kept shaking her head. "Fräulein Charlotte," Garp said. "She was Herr Doktor Thalhammer's patient."

"He has lots of patients," said the iron-gray maiden. She was consulting a list, but Garp did not know Charlotte's real name. Finally, he could think of no other way to identify her.

"The whore," he said. "She was a whore." The gray woman regarded him coolly; if Garp could detect no satisfaction in her expression, he could detect no sympathy either.

"The prostitute is dead," the old nurse said. Perhaps Garp only imagined that he heard a little triumph in her voice.

"One day, Meine Frau," he said to her, "you will be dead, too" [2, p. 117].

John Irving

Only the very rich in America can afford what those in lesser developed countries have as a matter of normal course: personal attention around the deathbed. In our technocratic society, medical care of the sick and dying has made unprecedented technological advances. However, in our fast-paced, increasingly heterogeneous, modern civilization, cultural and social support systems to care for the

---

[1]It is not difficult to recognize how indifferent the bustling activities of the world and its people are to the *private experiences* of human grief. I remember back to when my brother was killed. I received a call from a stranger informing me of the accident, was told he was dead by a stranger at the hospital, and wandered out of the emergency room onto the street where people were busily shopping, waiting for the movies, and swiftly driving to and fro about their business. In the cloudiness of my grief, even at that point, I remember thinking how private grieving has become and how isolated it is from the heroic-neon-light activity of everyday living. The words of Camus loom so relevant.

dying have not kept pace with technological advances. In this way then, the modern day deathbed, while techologically sophisticated, is visibly void of cultural ritual and ceremony and the regular, ongoing presence of human community.

As already noted, dying has become a social evil that is culturally denigrated and extraneous to the meaning sets of modern civilization. In this framework of cultural devaluation of dying and death, the dying process is not supported and sustained through stabilized patterns of ceremony, ritual, and fellowship. In addition, the nature of human community and shared concerns at the deathbed are reflective of the nature of community in society at large. The way Americans live, in or out of fellowship, will largely shape and define the way we die, in or out of fellowship. In this chapter, I will be exploring the theme of society and fellowship as it pertains to the human condition of dying patients.

THE NON-COMMUNAL ENVIRONMENT

One of the most salient features of life in America today is a decline in the spirit of community and a heightening of detached individualism.

As Nisbet observes in *The Sociological Tradition* and *The Quest for Community* [3, 4], the historical development of western society was intimately associated with the rise of political and social individualism. The certainties and unquestioned norms that characterized humanity's traditional ties to religious, kinship, and class structures before the French and Industrial Revolutions, have perceptibly disintegrated in the modern Western social setting. More importantly, no new societal patterns have arisen to provide the moral certainty of the traditional folkways and mores. As Nisbet comments:

> The historic triumph of secularism and individualism has presented a set of problems that looms large in contemporary thought. The modern release of the individual from traditional ties of class, religion, and kinship has made him free; but, on the testimony of innumerable works in our age, this freedom is accompanied not by the sense of creative release but by the sense of disenchantment and alienation. The alienation of man from historic moral certitudes has been followed by the sense of man's alienation from fellow man [4, p. 10].

The theme of alienation, as expressed by cultural images of loneliness, isolation, and the shallowness of relationships, is widely articulated in contemporary academic and popular literature. Indeed, serious novelists such as Camus, Kafka, Sartre, Hesse, and Greene on to more popular writers as King, Rossner and Roth, emphasize the splintering of humanity, the meaninglessness of relationships and the solitariness of modern living. Many recent films made for television and the cinema have also focused on the theme of the turmoil and disintegration of relationships. And, as one surveys the past two or three decades of scholarly activity, it becomes evident that the idea and hypothesis of alienation has assumed a central place in social science thought and research. It is not difficult to see, from these academic and popular indicators, that the drift of our times is away from stability in relationships and human fellowship.

In their attempt to study the implications of heightening individualism and alienation, Weiss and his colleagues have delineated four kinds of relationships which are essential to successful adjustment to the patterns of modern living and to the development of a personal sense of wellness [5, pp. 38-40]. First, it is important to know people who share our concerns. The function of this relationship is social integration; its absence leads to social isolation. Second, we need to know people we can depend on in a pinch. This relationship fulfills the need for social assistance, without which we feel anxious and vulnerable. Third, we need one or more close friends, individuals with whom we can be emotionally intimate, not people who are merely companions or acquaintances. These friendship relationships serve the vital function of fulfilling personal needs for intimacy, without which we would be left emotionally isolated and lonely. Fourth, it is essential to know one or more people who respect our competence. These respectful relationships bolster our self esteem; their absence leaves us feeling blemished and inadequate.

The point which Weiss and others before and since his study make is that the cultural framework and institutional organization of American society inhibits the regular, ongoing fulfillment of these relationship needs. The detached alienation of our age has promoted the growth of individualism, independence, and an unprecedented sense of *uninvolvement*, creating a social environment which makes it difficult to regularly fulfill the requirements of Weiss' needs. In some ways in these detached and uninvolved times, some forms of activism are on the increase, but most often these are increasingly characterized as ideologically based, single-interest groups and/or individuals and groups committed to the promotion of narrowly defined interests. The growing American involvement with narrowly defined, sometimes trivial issues, may be useful in providing individuals with an important sense of personal involvement with issues which seem manageable. Involvement with these kinds of issues enables the individual to feel he or she belongs to something and generates a sense of potency for the individual. However, it needs to be remembered that the forms of this type of involvement are consistent with the ethics of individualism and self-expression. They also point to *the generalized lack of involvement in* commonweal issues and the diminishment of collectively shared concerns among the American citizenry.

Again, as I have been emphasizing, the individual is left to his or her own abilities to carve out a web of satisfying relationships and a sense of purpose to living (and dying). The direction of this process of social change may be seen as a potentially liberating force creating important and unparalleled opportunities for the expression of human freedom and responsibility. On the flip side of the issue lies the fact that a widespread, stable base of social support is vanishing from the landscape of American society, exacerbating anxieties and vulnerabilities for the modern individual. And this has special and penetrating implications for the life experiences of dying individuals.

DYING AND LOSS OF FELLOWSHIP

The image of a person dying in a hospital room, surrounded by tubes, machines, and professional staff, is logically consistent with the broader American framework of bureaucratization, specialization, technologization, individualism, and alienation. In the modern scenario, as it is not unusual for Americans to live lives that are touched by loneliness, it is similarly not unusual for Americans to die alone and lonely.

In the first place, the individuals who largely shape, define, and dominate the process of dying, namely physicians, are generally not capable of providing and participating in support systems of intimacy and fellowship for the dying person. Two salient factors are relevant here. First, the organization and definition of work in the hospital setting emphasize technical medical-nursing care, and the structure of professional activity of doctors (and nurses as well) inhibits the regularized and accountable provision of "comfort work" [6]. The rational, technological framework of the organization of medical work stymies the formation of community and fellowship rituals that provide comfort and solace for the dying. Second, being restricted by the technological canons of professional training and detachment, physicians are structurally and psychically constrained from attending to the intimacy and fellowship needs of their dying patients.

It is also difficult for family and friends to attend satisfactorily to the human needs of dying people. In light of the absence of a collectively shared meaning set which makes sense of dying, it becomes understandably difficult for friends, family and patients to establish a stable and consistent pattern of mutual support. It is also difficult for the non-dying, who have lived much of their lives isolated from death-related concerns, to be able to empathize fully with the suffering and experiences of dying people. Finally, in this age of individualism, with the absence of shared concerns, it is increasingly normative for individuals to bring *their own*, well intentioned, definition of the situation to their interaction with dying patients. This absence of a shared set of definitions, understandings, and meanings can contribute to a feeling of polarization among those being personally touched by dying experiences. One patient speaks of how conflict can emerge, as she comments on how differently she and her mother see her situation:

> She has a terrible habit that annoys me. When we meet someone who has cancer, she always says: "Oh, your cancer is not as bad as his!" Like I should be thankful for having this kind of cancer. I know she is saying it for my own good—to make me feel better—but for me, any cancer is lousy, and I'm not able to handle it no matter how good of a . . . quote: how "good" of a cancer it may be.

> That irritates me. Oh, does that make me angry, and she cannot understand why I hate it when she does this.

This patient and her mother are responding to the problem of cancer and dying in radically different ways. The implications of the illness are also quite different for each. The patient is losing her self, her life, and her future, while her mother is losing her daughter and part of her motherhood. In the absence of a shared, cultural meaning set, grieving individuals are left to their own adaptive strategies in coping with dying. Such strategies will normatively be defined by one's own personality and particularized role position in relation to the dying experience. In this way, the sharing of concerns and its associated sense of social integration are tenuous and difficult to achieve for the dying person.

The divergence of concerns between doctor and patient is even more apparent as the technical orientation of medicine often conflicts with personal concerns of dying patients. Another patient speaks with painful candor:

> If I had a classroom of students in front of me, the one message I would tell them is to stay away from medicine. It won't help them in the long run, and it could care less about them as human beings . . .
>
> Why don't they have any compassion for the patient? All they do is continue to put me on new medications which they know won't work. They do this for themselves, not for me. They just don't care.

Three days later the same patient adds:

> The hair on my face. That's one thing I'll never forgive him [the oncologist] for. He knew that it was going to do this to my face. But he didn't care. He didn't care what it would mean to me as a person. I won't forgive myself, either, for letting him talk me into taking the medicine.

The irony illustrated by the above commentary is that advancements in technology and commitment to the use of technology in patient care are placing physicians in an irreconcilable dilemma with an important dimension of the Hypocratic Oath: PRIMUM NON NOCERE—Above all, do no harm. Furthermore, the managment of terminal illness through the application of medical technology may often conflict with the needs, desires, and hopes of patients. This conflict, which is a conflict between the doctor's narrow technical priorities and the patient's broad spectrum of human needs, is a drama that has been popularized by a number of celebrated cases and national media attention (Karen Ann Quinlan, "Whose Life is it Anyway?," etc.). But on a less celebrated and more ubiquitous plane, these conflicts regularly unfold in the everyday treatment of dying patients. They represent a clash of competing interests between and among doctors, family members, patients, lawyers, hospital administrators and even ethicists. In this manner, the modern, technical dying scenario is characterized by an absence of shared concerns. The result aggravates the social isolation of dying patients and in certain ways establishes a pluralistic dying model in which every death becomes individualized.

The lack of shared cultural meanings and the social realities of American society conspire against the continuing presence of family, friends, and community at the deathbed. In a society where dying, death, and suffering have become marginal phenomena, excluded from the course of daily social living, it is burdensome for individuals to feel at ease with and become active participants in the dying experience of another person. One family member speaks of the difficulty in watching and being with her dying husband throughout the course of his sufferings:

> The physical pain, that I can understand. But the hallucinations—the semiconscious writhing, which is more comfortable for him—is impossible for me. It's incredibly senseless. I can make more sense out of the physical pain than I can out of emotional suffering. Just watching him . . . I get so I can't take it, so I find myself making excuses for staying away. And then the guilt starts . . .

I hasten to emphasize, at this point, that the patient is not the only one isolated from interpersonal systems of support. Those who are personally involved with the dying person often find themselves in the situation of coping with their grief in isolation, with little assistance beyond their own personal abilities and resources.

In the context of medicalized dying and the absence of shared meanings, family members often become frustrated, helpless, and uninvolved spectators of the dying process of their loved ones. First of all, there is a lack of readily available and culturally approved norms to guide family members in their interactions with dying patients. As such, it is understandable that family members often feel confused and vulnerable in the presence of their dying loved one. One family member, speaking in the presence of and for her father and siblings, questions her mother's physician: "Should we talk to her? What should we say? What should we do when here? We are just so afraid of not doing the right thing."

As patients become visibly sicker, and as sufferings and deterioration become more evident, family feelings of helplessness correspondingly increase. The dying experience of the above patient, whose family expressed concern over how to relate to her, provides a useful illustration. The patient's disease was progressing steadily, and she began to complain: "I feel so confused. Oh, God. Oh, God. I just feel so confused."

It was believed that the patient's tumor had spread to her brain and that the source of her confusion was related to this progression of her disease. Her sense of confusion continued to the point where, several days after her initial complaints of disorientation, she lost awareness of herself and her situation. When her physician asked her to respond to some basic questions as what the year is, when her birthday is, who the president is, etc., she offered the following answers:

Today is January 4, 1981.[2] My home is _____ hospital. Today's date? 1974! I was born in 1973. The president? . . . Uh, the president?? Uh . . .

The patient continued to be confused and disoriented, signaling her dissatisfaction and frustration through verbal and physical expressions such as clenched fists, moans, and groans, depicting intense attempts at concentration and squirming in her bed. Excerpts from conversations with her physician on the following two days further illuminate her condition:

Doctor: Do you need anything tonight?
Patient: Yes. [nodding emphatically]
Doctor: What can I get for you?
Patient: I don't know, but something . . .

The physician, who saw that the patient was not requesting something specific but was grasping for some transcendence and control over her condition, offered her some words of reassurance and then left her (alone) to proceed on his rounds. The conversation resumed the following day:

Doctor: How are you doing today, Mrs. _____?
Patient: Not good.
Doctor: What's wrong?
Patient: I don't know. Oh boy . . . oh man, oh man . . . [she squirms in discomfort but not in pain and tosses her head side to side on her pillow]

As the patient became sicker during the final phase of her illness and displayed greater signs of distress and unease, her family was less and less present at her bedside. At the beginning of her final admission into the hospital, her husband, son, daughters, and mother-in-law were consistently present during visiting hours. But, as her disease and its physical/behavioral manifestations progressed, family visits became less regular. The pain of watching a loved one suffer, without a shared sense of purpose to the suffering, coupled with the inability to alleviate the suffering, is understandably a difficult burden to bear. In this vein, the family's absence from the dying process should not be immediately interpreted as a lack of concern or love, but rather it should be seen as a consequence of the helplessness, meaninglessness, and absence of social support systems which characterize the contemporary hospital deathbed scenario.

The "case" came to its conclusion at 10:15 one Friday morning. The resident walked into the patient's room to examine her and found her dead. (She had died alone.) After performing the technical ritual of certifying that she was dead, the resident called the attending physician's office to inform him of the patient's death and said: "Mrs. _____ has just died. What shall we do with the body?" The attending physician responded that the husband would be contacted

---

[2] It was actually mid-summer of another year.

and that he would then pass on the husband's wishes.[3] The body remained on the same floor, in a semi-private room with the bed curtains drawn, for over three hours while the attending physician tried to reach the patient's husband. The husband, who was finally contacted at his field assignment from work, was told over the phone that his wife had died earlier in the day.

The helplessness of those personally involved with the dying patient often leads to avoidance of contact with the patient or to normless, inconsistent, and anxious moments of interaction with the dying patient.

The isolation and the longing of the dying patient for support leads the patient to look to his or her doctor for comfort and reassurance. But, as we have seen, physicians' typical definition of professional obligations excludes them from providing deep and regular support for the psychosocial needs of dying patients. Despite the fact that doctors, especially detached-sympathetic-support doctors, do engage in comfort work, the amount and depth of comfort that physicians are able to provide is delimited by their technical role definition. The result of doctors' limited role definitions and the broad base of psychosocial needs of dying patients is that patients often feel neglected and abandoned by their doctors. One patient confides:

> I don't have full confidence in Dr. _____. He's a kind man and probably a good physician, but I don't have full confidence in him. I feel that he doesn't listen to me. He's always joking around and telling me what I should be doing, but he never listens to me.
>
> I can never count on him either. Whenever I really need him, he's never around. He just has this lady doctor see me, and I don't like her. Whenever there is a crisis, he's never around . . . off sailing or on vacation somewhere, but never where I need him.

The patient's doctor had been away at a medical convention when these comments were made. The physician returned from his conference three days later and during the course of his normal rounds entered into the patient's room to examine her. Upon seeing him, the patient perked up and exclaimed:

Patient: You deserted me! I'm sick all this time, and you do nothing to help me.

Doctor: [calmly smiling] What's the matter, don't I love you anymore? [Patient becomes very agitated, disturbed by the doctor's response, sighs, gives the doctor a dissatisfied look, and drops the issue.]

The patient, later in the same day, comments:

> See, what did I tell you? He's always ready with his jokes, so he doesn't have to listen to what I want to say.

Physicians are neither trained nor believe that they should function to fulfill the social assistance needs of patients. Patients, however, perhaps because of the

_____

[3] The medical staff had hoped to get an autopsy.

overwhelming desperation which can associate with dying, look to their physicians as they seek to have these needs fulfilled. Some doctors are markedly more caring than others in the care that they render, but whatever psychosocial support is given by the doctor is of a self-expressive, informal nature. Because of the way in which doctors' professional role definition is circumscribed by detachment and a technological focus, physicians are incapable of providing authentic personal and social support that would assist patients through their dying process.

There are also individuals in our society who die largely in isolation from other people because their families are dispersed throughout the country or because their family ties have seriously eroded. In addition, there are structural constraints inhibiting fellowship formation even for those dying patients who are connected to a network of people who care about them. The limitations of visiting hours, the restricting of children, the fact that the patient is in the hospital and not home, all serve as inhibitors to the formation of fellowship and community at the deathbed. But perhaps even more important is the fact that life responsibilities of family and friends continue on, unaffected by the circumstances of dying. Ariès and Camus were correct when they noted that society does not pause for dying or death. The realities of life with their professional, economic, personal, family, and social obligations limit the role that even the most dedicated of friends and family can play in providing support and comfort to the dying.

In an important sense, friends and family *visit* a dying person in the hospital; that is to say, they are *outsiders* who temporarily come to offer support, but they are not an integral presence in the everyday, moment-to-moment life of the terminally-ill patient. One patient reflects:

> I realize how much my husband means to me when he is not present. I get to missing him terribly, and I get to feeling sad, feeling loneliness. I know he won't be able to come again till tomorrow . . .

Another adds:

> I don't know what happened to my wife, who was supposed to come and visit. My son was also supposed to come to see me. Neither came, and I didn't know what to do.

In describing their perceptions of support and the absence thereof, despite many different types of personal circumstances, dying patients commonly and consistently bemoan the loneliness of evenings and of the night, especially sleepless nights.

Regardless of the efforts exerted by family and friends to be present[4] at the bedside of a dying loved one, and because of the organization of medicalized

---

[4] It is ironic that the one family member who was most dedicated to his dying relative (he was present every day during her repeated and sometimes extensive hospitalizations) was informed by his own physician that if he kept up his present regimen of caring for his wife, he himself would be dead in six months. This person was advised by his physician to have his wife placed in a nursing home.

dying and the individualism that forcefully drives everyday American activities, dying patients often live in the void and pain that results from inadequate or incomplete fulfillment of Weiss' needs. A vivid illustration comes to mind. It involves a seventy-year-old patient who had developed a tendency to drift in and out of states of irrationality. Her physicians had feared that her cancer had finally spread to her brain and was responsible for causing her hallucinations. Of particular importance, however, is that even when the patient was lucid, she had strong remembrances of the torments of her hallucinations. I walked into her room to see her and found her sitting up in bed, alone, trembling and crying. She had just awakened from a dream and was recounting how its images and themes had been coming to haunt her regularly since the problems with her hallucinations began a few days earlier:

> . . . the funeral velvet—that black draped all over the room. The incredibly kooky stuff that was going on. Behind the mirror, there are performers —dancing. You can't see them, but I can. The nurse, she is with them. I wouldn't take a pill from her. It scares me. It's all so irreligious. I don't believe in that stuff . . . I'm so afraid they are going to get my husband . . . they're going to make me die. A tall man came in, dressed in black, and told me I'm going to die. And there's a paper menorah in the corner of the room. . . .

The patient's vulnerabilities to her growing and hitherto unexplained periods of consuming but remembered irrationality, were exacerbated by her aloneness and loneliness. During the episode I sat with her for quite a while, holding her hand and just offering some reassurances. (But I myself was out of character. After all, I was present for the purpose of doing research on death and dying, not for providing social support.[5]) The patient was awaiting the arrival of her only regular visitor, her husband, who was expected in several hours. Until that time and even when he arrived, however, the patient would have to find ways of surviving her fears and vulnerabilities, in large part drawing on her own resources and adaptive strategies.[6]

Thus, at a time when individualism and alienation have become societal norms there is an obvious absence of culturally sanctioned meanings to the dying process. The sense of helplessness, abandonment, and isolation which surround the modern dying experience is a logical extension of the social forces of everyday living. The absence of and inadequacy of support systems to sustain people during the grief of dying and the deficient fulfillment of Weiss' needs increasingly isolate the dying person in a *privatized world of survival and coping*. This in turn helps to initiate a self-fulfilling prophecy of making dying increasingly meaningless and tragic. The result is that it becomes ever more difficult to

---

[5] For a useful discussion of the spectrum of roles that a fieldwork-researcher typically assumes in the course of medical ethnographies, see: Charles Bosk. "The Fieldworker as Watcher and Witness." *Hasting Center Report*. June, 1985, pp. 10–14.

[6] Her physicians were reluctant to treat her hallucinatory symptoms for fear that this would mask other symptoms relevant to their treatment of her cancer.

establish and sustain the presence of human community at the deathbed. In this way, the process and sufferings of dying are becoming increasingly privatized, and the privatizing of the dying experience has become a salient means of managing and controlling the death process.

REFERENCES

1. A. Camus, *The Plague*, Vintage Books, New York, 1972.
2. J. Irving, *The World According to Garp*, E. P. Dutton, New York, 1978.
3. R. Nisbet, *The Sociological Tradition*, Basic Books, New York, 1966.
4. —————, *The Quest for Community*, Oxford University Press, New York, 1981.
5. R. Weiss, The Fund of Sociability, *Transaction*, July/August 1969.
6. A. Strauss, *Social Organization of Medical Work*, University of Chicago Press, Chicago, 1985.

CHAPTER
5

Modern Dying and Social Organization of the Hospital

The final medical solution to human problems: remove everything from the body that is diseased or protesting, leaving only enough organs which— by themselves, or hooked up to appropriate machines—still justify calling what is left of the person a "case"; and call the procedure "humanec- tomy" [1, p. 70].

Thomas Szasz

Since the introduction of modern technology, the hospital has lost its aura of being a place of comfort and has instead become an establishment resembling a factory, where illnesses are taken care of, rather than human beings [2, p. 22].

Henry Heinemann

A hospital is a bureaucratically organized social institution whose function is to treat and heal disease. The management of disease is approached through a tech- nological and scientific orientation which emphasizes the priorities of rationality and efficiency. According to institutional justifications of the medical point of view, rationalization and standardization of care and depersonalization of pa- tients are "worth the price" when medical results benefit the patient. The under- lying premise of the hospital's organization of medical care is consistent with the central motivational values of the technological consciousness, namely, that the vital needs of human beings are reducible to technologically manageable com- ponents. Therefore, in the hospital scheme of things, the requirements of a pa- tient's humanity yield to medical means of technical analysis, carried out by specialists possessing certain impenetrable skills which translate patient needs into a series of management procedures and regimens. According to this philos- ophy of medical care, if a problem does not have an objective, somatic base and a technical solution, then it is not a real problem worthy of real attention.

The bureaucratic ethos by which the hospital organizes its daily activities serves an important function in sustaining the technical detachment of a physi- cian from the psychosocial needs of the dying. As Weber discusses, the coordin- ating principles of specialization and rationalization allow for the regular and uninterrupted fulfillment of the duties legislated by the bureaucracy [3, p. 196].

The bureaucratic environment of the hospital continually impresses on the physician the role expectations of detachment, emotional neutrality and objectivity that were spawned during the formative years of medical education. This is useful in maintaining the objective-technical base of the doctor's training throughout the years of professional practice and in reducing the obstructive presence of subjectivity, irrationality and emotionality in the everyday structure of the hospital. As Berger puts it, the primary effect of bureaucratic consciousness in technological civilization is the management of emotionality [4, p. 57]. In this way, when emotions are expressed by patients, family members, etc., they are defined foremost as inappropriate and the physician is legitimately able to respond in a manner which ignores those outbreaks and restricts or inhibits further emotional expressions. This observation becomes clear in the following scenario. A doctor was on the course of his daily rounds, being followed by seven first-year students who had been assigned to him for one afternoon a week, for six weeks, in a program on "perspectives in patient care." The doctor encountered in the hallway the spouse of a middle-aged woman whose tests had recently come back from the lab with a diagnosis of myeloma in an advanced stage. The spouse wanted to talk to the doctor, who was quite willing to do so. The doctor and his entourage proceeded into a treatment room which would allow some privacy. The physician told the patient's husband the facts of the case: that his wife had a serious form of cancer and that her life expectancy was about one to two years. The husband began to cry and continued to cry during the six to seven minutes of conversation with the doctor. The husband was insisting that the doctor lie to his wife about her condition; the doctor was refusing saying, "I have to tell her she has cancer, but we don't have to let her know how bad it is." The doctor very calmly, rationally, and *without any recognition of or attention to the husband's emotional outpourings*, convinced him that his wife should be told of the cancer, but that the emphasis in the discussion would be on treatment modalities. The nature of this interaction is humanly fascinating and notable but fairly standard for the bureaucratic interactional processes which typify doctor-patient communications. Thus, what would have been virtually impossible in an ordinary social interaction, namely, proceeding as if the emotional expressions of the husband did not exist at all, was fully supported by the bureaucratic organization of patient care. In this way, the emotional turbulence of dying was severely restricted by the bureaucratic-technical focus of the physician. And, what an introduction to detachment and objectivity these first-year students received!

The hospital-based system of medical care is also a reflection of and contributor to the growing specialization of the medical profession. Doctors treating only certain types of conditions, others exclusively involved in narrow technical activities, e.g., reading x-rays and CT scans, interns rotating from area to area or patient to patient, nurses increasingly becoming identified with a specified area of care such as pediatrics or oncology, are all reflective of the hierarchical and specialized division of labor that characterizes the structure of medical care in the hospital:

> ... the trend is clear; increasing numbers of physicians are seeking the personal security and satisfaction of specialization.... To be able to deliver what he knows is the best, the doctor today is forced to limit the breadth of his practice—to specialize [5, p. 681].

As specialization becomes an institutionalized norm, a vast array of technical and medical experts become essential to the staffing of a modern hospital. The irony of this situation is that comprehensiveness in medical care is defined through an inward spiral of reductionist activity, increasing circumscription of professional orientation and competency, and the distancing from breadth. In the framework of specialization, the idea of TOTALITY becomes operational through the independent functioning of isolated units of technical activity. David Mechanic summarizes the importance of the compartmentalization and specialization of care in the bureaucratic milieu of the hospital:

> Within the technical scientific organization, chief consideration is given to the means to achieve most efficiently a high level of diagnostic work. In this setting, medical assessment is highly specialized, on the assumption that experts in particular fields are more knowledgeable than a general doctor. Moreover, time units are developed which allow adequate evaluation to take place, without sacrificing the efficiency of the doctors output. ... The patient thus becomes a unit which is moved from department to department, so that each can exercise its specialized function with dispatch and efficiency. Each department views the patient in terms of its specialized function, giving highest priority to its particular task [6, p. 170-171].

In direct correlation with the degree to which the patient is narrowly defined and considered, the task of the physician becomes commensurately narrow and standardized. Inherently then, emotional needs of the patient are excluded from the specialized, standard, technical purview of the hospital organization of medical care. The growing tendency for specialization in patient care has also, ironically, become intertwined with the societal movements against fragmentation and toward self-expression. As already discussed, the hospice movement is seeking to implement a broader, more integrated spectrum of patient care than the compartmentalized program of care offered by the hospital. The establishment of hospice programs in America, however, is consistent with the modern societal and medical tendency toward specialization. The hospice as an alternative to the hospital is a highly specialized institution, which caters to needs of a highly specific population, namely, terminally-ill patients. The hospice has established new and specialized professional roles of caring for the dying, namely, hospice medical director, hospice chaplain, hospice nurses, and hospice volunteers. In this way the hospice, while seeking a more comprehensive approach to patient care, is still situated within the broader framework of specialization and compartmentalization of care.

Given this introduction to the bureaucratic blueprint of hospital-based care, I will now turn attention to exploring the hospital as a system of dehumanization for the medical patient in general and the dying person in particular.

THE HOSPITAL AS A TOTAL INSTITUTION

Every social institution is capable of dominating the time, interests and activities of people in it. Some institutions obviously have greater capacity in this regard than others. A total institution represents the pinnacle of this dominating capacity and is generally characterized by physical separation from and the blocking of continuous social intercourse with the outside world [7]. A hospital, although not completely separational, isolates its patients from the outside world and generally separates the control of patient activity from patient, family, and community influence. Although the capacity and tendency for domination may not exist unchallenged, as we saw in Kesey's *One Flew Over the Cuckoo's Nest* and as reflected by some of the patient experiences in this book, the organizational thrust of the hospital is towards standardization, routinization, and objectification—that is to say, towards control and management.

Goffman's discussion of total institutions depicts not just how efficient the physical and social organization for totality is in accomplishing a multitude of tasks, but also the potential for dehumanization of the forms of life that are administered by total institutions. A main focus of *Asylums* is how a person's self is sociologically structured through the total institutional living experience. In many ways, an individual's self is changed and "mortified" upon entrance into the total institution. This is accomplished through a variety of strategies, policies, and techniques which define and redefine a person's self-concept into a set of behavioral expectations and requirements that facilitate the bureaucratic operation and flow of work. Entrance into a hospital or other institution entails a standardized procedure for processing, identifying, and labelling personhood. A process of role disengagement which transforms the incoming person into an admitted patient is initiated by the interactions that take place between admitting staff and the patient. I have heard patients regularly complain about excessive waiting for admissions procedures to be completed; the nature of these interactions being governed by the operational needs of the bureaucracy (insurance information, etc.). The perceptive patient knows that he or she is being processed by hospital workers in ways that emphasize objective, standardized considerations.

The initial moments of socialization on the wards of the hospital further give the patient the understanding that the hospital routine is largely interested in individuals only as patients. Although staff normatively "welcome" the patient with pleasant conversation and do often informally chat with patients whom they know, the stage is being set for starting the operating engines of the bureaucratic patient-management process. Nurses and residents will take extensive case histories and perform preliminary medical exams (having sent for and received charts from past hospitalizations). At this point, the wheels of the bureaucracy are quickly set in motion: the family is isolated from the care of the patient, and the authority of nurses, interns and residents is established. The attending or admitting physician is generally not present during this period of initiation, but when he or she visits the patient later in the day on rounds, the patient is given a comprehensive physical exam, called a "work-up." The work-up includes a hands-on physical exam, some of which has already been performed by the intern or resident, asking a comprehensive set of questions relevant to physical symptomatology and disease management, identifying what tests need to be done, ordering medications to be administered, and establishing and informing the patient of the plan of treatment that is being designed.

After a mere eight hours or so, if the patient was unaware of or had forgotten about the requirements of the patient role, he or she learns that deference, obedience and compliance are required. The patient, even if responded to in the most sensitive and humane patterns of care, is still defined by and through the work requirements of the staff's professional role obligations. As Mr. Smith becomes transformed into "Mr. Smith—The Cancer Patient in 402," the uniqueness, feelings and human expressions of the personal side of the patient become reduced to anecdotal significance.

When patients are admitted to a hospital for the treatment of serious, life-threatening disease, their primary concern is with matters of life and death significance. However, as their concerns, which are seen as private and personal, are immersed within the confines of a purely technological definition of patient care, the expression of the individual's haunting worries about the possibility of dying are effectively circumscribed. The person's anxiety over the possibility of dying is redefined into less threatening, more manageable categories of patient care. That is to say, the broad issue of dying becomes condensed and packaged into a series of patient management procedures, a series of tests, diagnoses, medical and surgical interventions, etc. Thus, the very human and potentially meaningful expressions of anger, vulnerability, fear, and emotional turbulence that characterize a personalized response to dying are rendered insignificant through the standardized objectification of a patient's identity. Dying is denied, or more correctly, it is organized and contained by the bureaucratic underpinnings of total institutional social interactions.

The objectification of personhood is functional from the point of view of medical efficiency. Any patient or family member who fails to accept the institution's definition of proper behavior interferes with the felicitous carrying out of work tasks. One woman who was deeply embittered at the grimness of her husband's prognosis for melanoma became aggressively confrontational with her husband's attending physician. She indicted and criticized the care he had been receiving and was complaining about the lack of commitment (or her perceptions thereof) to her husband's full recovery. The attending physician, tiring of her attitude, asked her to "please wait in the hallway" so he could begin his work-up of the patient. She refused, saying, "No! _____ (referring to her husband) doesn't mind me being here." The doctor, believing that the woman was a threat to the efficient and standardized carrying out of his work task, informed her that unless she waited outside her husband would not be examined. After an emotionally charged confrontation, the doctor's require-ment prevailed, and she reluctantly left for the hallway. (The patient meanwhile had been lying on his bed, clad only in his underpants, quietly watching the interaction for the full five minutes it took.) Another patient, who had read just about every piece of research in the medical journals that was pertinent to his case,[1] became defiant of his doctor's medical strategies. He would engage his physicians in time-consuming discussions about the relative merits of differ-ent courses of treatment. He was remarkably conversant and knowledgeable about studies in the cancer journals, but his efforts to design his own plan of treatment were dismissed as "inappropriate and ridiculous" by his physicians. The patient was told by his two doctors that either he complied with their program of treatment for him, or he should find himself another hospital. (And the latter is precisely what happened.)

It is scenarios such as these which become disruptive to the smooth flow of the doctor's work task and to the standardized operation of the medical bureaucracy. Expressions of individuality can be tolerated only if they do not interfere with the technological routine of patient care. The total institutional framework of the hospital accomplishes this task by defining the concerns of patients, particularly dying patients, into a rational and objective definition of reality which transmutes the social self of the patient into a "non-person medical entity." Goffman eloquently describes this process as:

> ... the wonderful brand of "non-person" treatment found in the medi-cal world, whereby the patient is greeted with what passes as civility and said farewell to in the same fashion with everything in between going on as if the patient weren't there as a social person at all, but only as a possession that someone has left behind [7, pp. 341–342].

As we can see, the observations of Goffman are still remarkably relevant twenty years later.

This reductionist definition of medical care is responsible for the many abuses and the neglect of the personal and social needs of patients. One afternoon, for example, I walked into a semi-private room of four patients to see one of the terminally-ill patients in my study. In the bed immediately to the left of the door-way, a man with testicular cancer was undergoing a preoperative examination

_____
[1] A common piece of backstage humor about this patient among doctors was the state-ment: "When he dies you can have his money, I'll take his medical library."

and questioning by two surgical residents. As the doctors were examining the patient (actually, one examined him while the other sat at the foot of the bed and took notes), it became clear that these young surgeons were interested exclusively in the physical-technical considerations that were relevant to the upcoming operation. The patient was examined without the bed curtains being drawn, and the patient's physicality was displayed for any passerby to see, as his legs were spread and genitals fully exposed. I asked the attending oncologist of the patient I was seeing, who had also witnessed this scene, how he could tolerate such callous disregard for the dignity of the patient and not have said something to the residents about their behavior. The oncologist replied: "I would have said something if they had been medical residents, not surgical."

The social structure of the hospital is arranged on many of the principles that form a total institution, and the objective, fragmented world view that is promoted by the hospital creates an environment which is conducive even to extreme and obvious indicators of dehumanization. In addition, the idea of specialization and bureaucratization of care enables even perceptive, detached-sympathetic-support physicians to deny responsibility for structurally embedded abuses of patient care. Most significantly, the objectified realities of the structure of the hospital are largely capable of channeling the subjective, personal side of human dying into a medical category that is rationally and technically manageable. In this scheme of things, in that dying represents a *subjective* label that is attached to an objective disease state, dying becomes a non-existent process. In this way, the very idea of dying is "denied," that is to say, contained by the operational realities of the hospital. The well known comment by an intern interviewed by Elisabeth Kübler-Ross becomes readily understandable in this light: "There are no dying people here!"

PATIENT ALIENATION WITHIN THE HOSPITAL

Alienation has been variously defined by social scientists as a process which separates humanity from necessary and inherent qualities of being human. The idea of alienation becomes meaningful on a personal level when individuals find themselves living in societal circumstances which inhibit the fulfillment and attainment of those qualities that an individual perceives as important to the definition of his or her human identity.

One of the major limitations of the concept of alienation is that it is often used in academic and abstract ways which are divorced from ordinary, everyday human realities. I'm really not quite sure, despite all of the academically inspirational alienation literature that has been produced in the past twenty years or so, what it means on the level of ordinary human significance to say that humanity is being separated from "essential and inherent qualities that constitute the process of being human." There have been attempts made to address the issue of the applicability of the concept of alienation to human life and to operationalize the concept in ways that connect it to the plane of observable human reality. It is beyond the scope of this book to study these attempts and evaluate comprehensively the alienation literature. Nevertheless, I will utilize a number of measures of alienation found in the literature in order to explicate the value of the idea of alienation to the study of people dying within the total institutional confines of the hospital setting.

Powerlessness, or the notion that something cannot be done, is a salient indicator of alienation [8, pp. 784-785]. It refers to the belief of an individual that he or she cannot determine or influence a desired goal. It is best expressed by the feeling "there is not much I can do about the important personal and social problems confronting me."

The feeling of powerlessness may be induced by natural or artificial causes. In many circumstances it is in the very nature of being human that one is unable to affect important life issues. Powerlessness then results from the inherent fragility and vulnerability of the human species. Or, feelings of personal impotence in the face of important life events may be impressed on individuals by the values and institutions of society. In this way, human powerlessness is a structurally induced phenomenon of culturally specific circumstances. The alienation of dying patients in twentieth century America is a self-exacerbating blend of naturally and societally rooted powerlessness.

The unavoidability of dying afflicts every living species but the certainty of death has special implications for human beings. The nature of human reason and self awareness shackles humanity with the awareness of its fate and our inabilities in the face of this fate. As we have already discussed, great societal efforts to reduce the terror of death have been inspired by the ubiquitous absurdity that all rational human beings know that they and their loved ones someday must die. In this way then, it is in the nature of a human being to anticipate the loss of one's life, the loss of one's future, and the loss of important relationships. The anxieties associated with this process of separation form the basis of human anxiety and fear of death, according to Fromm [9]. The dying person feels and is threatened by the inevitable sense of loss that dying begets. The dying person also anticipates crossing over into the unknowable abyss that is death, and naturally wonders about what death means and brings. It is not unnatural in light of the human tenacity for life, that the anticipation of that fleeting moment or second, when one takes one's final breath never to breathe again, will shadow all of the loss and uncertainty of death with an identifiable sense of powerlessness.[2]

---

[2] It needs to be remembered that while the cultural rituals of traditional death patterns served to mitigate the powerlessness associated with death, the existence of these rituals and dramas of the deathbed, in and of itself, speaks of the natural powerlessness of human beings in the face of death and of the need for humanity to transcend this impotence individually and collectively.

In addition to natural powerlessness, artificially induced impotence abounds for the modern dying person. The sufferings of dying are intensified through modern cultural definitions and meaning sets. In that life is defined as a possession, modern society has produced an explicit image of death robbing us of something we own. Because the death of a loved one is mourned by a shrinking community, the process of grieving may be emotionally intensified for the diminishing circle of intimate family and friends. The intensification of grief coupled with the diminishment of support systems tends to exacerbate feelings of powerlessness for the dying person and his family. The bottom line is that despite the promises of technology, human vulnerability in the presence of death has ultimately changed very little. The faith that Americans place in science and technology, however, has created expectations of omnipotence within the American frame of mind. The result of these expectations is that feelings of powerlessness are made more acute when death comes knocking at our door.

There are several hazards of powerlessness relevant here. The human needs of the dying person are intensified at a time when support systems of solace and comfort have been diminished. Thus, when dying does present itself to one's personal doorstep, the ideal vision of living a life that is undisturbed by death is rent asunder. The pain of this disillusionment not only serves to make death and dying more emotionally pungent, but also threatens to unleash a barrage of individual and collective emotions expressing the modern absurdities of dying. The need for containment of these human responses to the cultural intensity of dying emerges, and it is the technological-bureaucratic management of the patient which fulfills this function rather well. As death is contained through the forces of technological manipulation, the individual becomes increasingly subjected to the controls of the medical bureaucracy. It seems that in view of the cultural definition and circumstances of dying, along with the attempt to contain the problem of death through technical management, like topsy, the powerlessness of dying patients grows and grows . . . as their disease progresses.

An important dimension of powerlessness, then, is a social construction of the non-person treatment imposed on dying individuals in the total institution of a hospital. Having had so much of their personal identity stripped away and diminished, dying persons become less and less capable of affecting and making decisions about their own fate. The facilitation of staff work activities demands passivity in the patient role. Otherwise, probing, poking, exploring, injecting medicines, etc., would not be the smoothly accomplished tasks that they are today, but would become precarious professional activities for the men and women of medicine. In addition, it is interesting to observe how many decisions about the life of a patient are made without seriously consulting the patient. Patients often are informed of the treatment they will be receiving in a manner that is more of an afterthought than anything else. As Cornelius Ryan descriptively tells in the autobiographical account of his battle with cancer, his doctors dismissed the importance of his need to be involved in decision making about his course of treatment:

> "Please tell me exactly what you have found," I said.
> "I think, Mr. Ryan, much of the findings are too technical to go into. I would prefer to explain this in my own way." . . .
> "Doctor," I began, "the technical findings concern me and my future. I'd very much appreciate your telling me what they are."
> He did not unbend.
> "You are a difficult man, Mr. Ryan, in your persistence in groping for details you could not possibly understand" [10, p. 84].

Goffman argues that the passification of the patient and the objectification of personhood so completely suppress a patient's personal presence that his or her fate can be openly discussed around the bedside by a variety of experts, without the experts having to feel undue concern. Presumably a technical vocabulary helps in this regard [7, p. 442]. There are, in the major medical centers, many structurally embedded patterns that wholly but temporarily decimate the humanity of a patient, e.g., medical and surgical rounds, grand rounds, and sitting in a wheelchair or lying on a stretcher in a hallway awaiting various diagnostic procedures. I have not observed the complete nullification of personhood of which Goffman speaks, as the presence and/or expression of patient and family dissatisfactions bring the personal presence of the patient to the fore. Nevertheless, regular and sustained strategies designed to contain disruptive and emotionally turbulent expressions of dying patients are largely present. In addition, the fact that physicians do separate backstage behavior from front stage interactions with patients, indicates that physicians are sensitive to the presence of the personal self of their patients, and by default, give recognition to the value of personhood.

The powerlessness of personhood is demeaning for any medical patient, but as Mechanic pointed out, there is at least some medical use-value associated with the objectification of the patient. The terminal patient by definition, however, cannot be expected to get well again. Thus, the dying patient is faced with suffering through the human indignities of the total institutional hospital while simultaneously not being able to receive the full benefits of modern medical technology, i.e., recovery. Dying patients become subjected to a double failure: the technical failure and inability of modern medicine to effect a cure along with a structurally rooted neglect of the requirements of their personal and social needs.

The central irony of the powerlessness of dying, however, becomes evident after just a few months of observation in the hospital setting: the more the bureaucratic system of care neglects and dehumanizes the patient, the more the patient is likely to become grateful to the agents of this dehumanization. The more the system operates to define the patient as an object to be managed through technical activities, the scarcer and hence more precious personal attention from nurses, physicians, and other technicians becomes. In the presence of this institutionally rooted scarcity, at a time when the emotional and social needs of patients are heightened by the demands of the dying experience, patients tend to become increasingly indebted to the medical staff for the routine and standardized version of care they provide. In this way, the more individual personhood is neglected, especially at such a vital and vulnerable time, the more the neglected person becomes appreciative of any source of attention to his or her individual needs.

The Orwellian underpinnings of the process of powerlessness are readily evident. In terms of moral and social principles, there is little difference between the powerlessness of dying in a total institutional setting and the impotence of individuals in Orwell's Oceania. Indeed, the similarities are striking. The citizenry of Oceania were controlled through rational and efficient use of technical means. Dying individuals in twentieth century America are defined and dominated by the technological foundations of contemporary medical practice. The inner party, the experts of social control, was in charge of implementing Orwell's fictitious society. The inner party, the experts of medical control, is in charge of managing the plight of dying people in the hospital setting. The power of the experts in Oceania was total; Winston and Julia's revolt was doomed from the very beginning. The power of the hospital system is not as encompassing as that found in Oceania, but the technical and bureaucratic rules, standards and norms of hospital life are the guiding principles that shape the experience of death in the modern hospital environment.

In the "Afterword" to *1984*, Erich Fromm relates Simone Weil's definition of power to Orwell's discussion of power and power relations in Oceania. Power, according to Weil, is the capacity to transform a person into a corpse, that is to say, into a thing [16, p. 263]. The point that Fromm advances is that Weil's idea of power accurately typifies power relations in everyday American life. More specifically relevant to considering the plight of dying patients, the power base of the modern, cosmopolitan hospital, with its technological omnipotence and authoritative medical healers, strains toward accomplishing the precise transformation of the human being that Weil described. The non-person treatment of the dying, the cadaver orientation of patient care, the bureaucratic organization of the hospital, and the restriction of the social presence of the patient for the benefit of technical activity have in fact reduced the dying patient to the status of a thing. The final consequence and means of dehumanization in *1984* was the systematic implantation of a sense of gratitude for the workings of the party and the system. It is difficult to forget the horror of the closing scene wherein Winston, sipping his Victory Gin contentedly, reflects on how everything was right with the world: He Loved Big Brother. Although the hospital system of patient care cannot effect the total domination of consciousness which we see in *1984*, there is a stringently enforced requirement that patients be grateful to and compliant with the directives of the benevolent inner party [12, p. 352].

In short, institutionally induced insignificance of the individual in the face of dying is the ultimate expression of the containment of the sociohuman dying experience and of the power of the technological orientation of the profession of medicine and of the broader cultural and social systems.

In important ways, my discussion of powerlessness has illustrated two other salient indicators of alienation: meaninglessness and social isolation. Meaning-lessness refers to an individual's sense of understanding the events in which he or she is engaged [8, p. 786]. It refers to a culturally bound feeling of confu-sion or frustration or "the sense that for some reason things have become so complicated in the world today that I really don't understand what is going on" [13, pp. 223-242]. As we have already seen, death is unmitigated in the modern setting, by rituals of support and culturally rooted meaning sets. The cultural labelling of dying as evil, exacerbated by medical neglect of sociohuman needs, makes the dying patient increasingly reliant and dependent upon techno-logical-curative intervention. However, perhaps for the first time in their lives, dying patients are finding that science and technology are failing to live up to their promises. The generalized faith which Americans place in science and technology becomes shaken at this point and the dying person understandably becomes dismayed and confused by his or her startling awareness of the limita-tions of the technological way of life. We have also seen evidence of the inter-actional normlessness that surrounds the dying patient and which contributes an overriding sense of confusion to the dying process. I have regularly observed and heard patients expressing turbulent exasperation over "why this had to happen to me." The structural realities of the hospital frame of reference and the broader cultural meaning sets which shape the realities of modern dying fail to adequately relieve and explain the patient's quandary, driving the senselessness of dying deeply into the life experience and perceptions of the dying patient. The specific consequences of alienation for the psychosocial identity of dying patients will be explored more fully in the following chapter as I portray the stigmatization and defilement of identity for dying human beings.

A third indicator of alienation has also been interwoven into the discussion. Social isolation refers to "the feeling of being lonely" [13, p. 227] or the yearning for the fulfillment of Weiss' needs. As already discussed, the social iso-lation of the dying is reflective of the individualism and diminishment of community in American life. The transfer of the place of death to the hospital, however, with its bureaucratic patterns of patient management further exasper-ates the isolation and the solitude of the dying patient. In a very straightforward way, the total institutional structure of the hospital care of dying patients de-emphasizes the priority of social integration and through insistence on following a course of treatment that is exclusively technical in orientation, the idea of social support becomes reduced to a superfluous afterthought.

The crucial issue which emerges is that of control. Dying patients today, due to culturally and socially inspired alienation, are increasingly faced with uncertainties and a shadow of normlessness that fills their dying days. The question of what should be done, when, where and how it should be done is normatively decided by physicians motivated by their technocratic consciousness, not patients. In addition, patients are increasingly placed into a situation where they are personally responsible for establishing some sense of meaning and purpose to their own dying. In this way, another paradox is created by the technological management of dying, in that at a time when patients are being held individually responsible for carving out meaning to their dying, the alienation of patients is at its height. The irony of having an increase in personal involvement with the private definition of dying being associated with increased detachment from cultural and social support systems of dying is explicitly consistent with the forces of technocracy and self-expressiveness which dominate life in America today.

The alienation of the patient and the institutionally based avoidance of death which I observed were less monolithic than that reported in the classic studies of Sudnow and Glaser and Strauss. Nevertheless, the overall impact of objectification of the patient and dehumanization of the social self is just as salient as it was during the time of these studies. In addition, the increasing normlessness, which I have reported, was not nearly as apparent twenty years ago. This normlessness has led to a sense of confusion and groping on the part of physicians for answers to difficult issues, which in and of itself has elicited the emergence of a variety of forms of detachment, alienation and avoidance. Indeed, many of the contemporary ways of avoiding and objectifying death are more intricate, subtle, and sophisticated, giving the appearance of a breakdown in the ethic of standardized, bureaucratic management of the dying. Underlying the emerging variation in form, however, are the rational and technically based coordination of activities that are the heart of any total institution. Thus, while some of the forms of the total institutional control over the dying process are changing, the substantive forces of alienation loom very large.[3]

One scenario that effectively illuminates my point entailed a middle-aged woman, with seriously advanced cancer, who was quickly approaching the moment of death. The woman was in a private room with an oxygen tent hookup to provide some help for her laborious breathing. She was in tremendous pain and discomfort and was becoming increasingly weak. Yet, in a strange way, despite her technological surroundings and physical debility, she looked very pretty. Her physician walked into her room during the course of his rounds and found her husband quietly sitting by her side. After an exchange of amenities, the physician sprang into a flurry of technical activity, listening to the woman's chest, probing her abdominal areas, checking the swelling in her lymph nodes,

---

[3] I should also note that, like Sudnow, I observed no instances whereby physicians offered comfort to family members, and in *every* case where conversation drifted towards death and dying, the idea of death was couched in a technical emphasis and language.

etc. During the course of this professional activity, he informed the patient and her husband that he was going to give her some medication for the pain.

The doctor left the room, indicating he wanted to give the medication by injection so that it would take effect more quickly. He promptly returned with the syringe and medicine and began to prepare the patient for an injection, only to find that her veins had collapsed. He searched fruitlessly for four to five minutes for a vein that would tolerate the injection and then informed the patient that a nurse would come down and administer the medicine by mouth. Assuring the patient that he would make every effort to keep her as comfortable as possible, the doctor took his leave. The patient's husband followed, about fifteen feet behind, out into the hallway and called to the doctor when both were fully out of the room and the door had swung closed.

There is no effective way to describe the husband's facial expressions except to say that he was lost, aching, lonely, confused, and desperate. During the course of a very brief conversation, tears swelled in his eyes, and he struggled to hold them back. He asked the doctor how his wife was doing and what could be expected. The physician very calmly responded: "I doubt she'll make it through the night." The husband, pleading and hoping with every ounce of faith his soul could muster, asked if there was anything else that could be tried. The physician calmly responded that there was nothing that could be done for her except to try to make her as comfortable as possible.

The conversation lasted for approximately two minutes, during which time no explicit mention of death was made nor was any attempt to recognize or comfort the husband's suffering made by the physician. Indeed, I did observe a noticeable straining on the part of the physician to exit from this death scene as quickly as possible. As I have already discussed, the tendency to flee from death typifies physician responses to the nearing of death. As one doctor expressed it, "the roller skates are put on," namely, one gets as quickly detached from the death setting as possible. As the physician bade farewell to the husband and turned to leave, I did the same. Upon glancing at the husband who was returning back to the room on the brink of tears, the meaning of alienation became so apparent. Sensing the powerlessness and loss of the husband, and thinking of his wife struggling for breath, awaiting his return to the bedside, I saw so clearly how deep their needs were and how miserably they remained unaddressed. To this day, I do not forgive myself for not eschewing my own professional role definition and the obligations I had for the remainder of the day, in order to stay with the patient and her husband during the final hours of her life.

Many of the ironies of dying in modern society to which I have pointed are made evident by this situation. All too often, dying patients and isolated pockets of loved ones are left to their own resources and strengths at a time when they are highly vulnerable and their personal and social selves have been reduced to a point of insignificance. In this sense, the factors of patient powerlessness are exacerbated at a time when the strength of personhood is most essential to any adequate pattern of coping. Although it is only implicit in the above scenario, the cultural and social meaninglessness of dying heightens feelings of vulnerability and impotence. A self-exacerbating, culturally unmitigated process of alienation defines the nature of dying in the bureaucratic social system that is the modern hospital.

The similarities between Sudnow's study and this one are remarkable. The important point, however, lies not so much in the respective affinity of the findings and interpretations, but rather in unveiling that despite twenty years of preoccupation with the study of death and dying spanning the two works, the "death work" which typifies the modern urban medical center has remained notably consistent over the years. It is in this way that, despite the extraordinary influx of books, editorials, journals, and media coverage of death and dying, the American approach to death remains moored within a framework of technological and bureaucratic control.

REFERENCES

1. T. Szasz, *The Second Sin*, Anchor Books, New York, 1974.
2. H. Heinemann, Human Values in the Medical Care of the Terminally Ill, in *Psychosocial Aspects of Terminal Care*, B. Schoenberg, et al., Columbia University Press, New York, 1972.
3. M. Weber, Bureaucracy, in *From Max Weber*, translated by Hans Gerth and C. W. Mills. Oxford University Press, New York, 1958.
4. P. Berger, et al. *The Homeless Mind: Modernization and Consciousness*, Random House, New York, 1973.
5. C. Code, Determinants of Medical Care: A Plan for the Future, *The New England Journal of Medicine, 283*:13, 1970.
6. D. Mechanic, *Medical Sociology*, The Free Press, New York, 1968.
7. E. Goffman, *Asylums*, Doubleday, New York, 1969.
8. M. Seeman, On the Meaning of Alienation, *Americal Sociological Review, 24*:6, 1959.
9. E. Fromm, *The Art of Loving*, Harper and Row, New York, Chapter One, 1956.
10. C. Ryan and K. M. Ryan, *A Private Battle*, Simon and Schuster, New York, 1979.
11. E. Fromm, Afterword, in G. Orwell, *1984*, Harcourt Brace Jovanovich, Inc., New York, 1949.
12. E. Shelp, Courage: A Neglected Virtue in the Patient-Physician Relationship, *Social Science and Medicine, 18*:4, 1984.
13. G. Zito, Marx, Durkheim and Alienation, *Social Theory and Practice, 3*:2, 1975.

CHAPTER 6

The Stigma of Dying

Man's nature, his passions, and anxieties are a cultural product [1, p. 27].

Erich Fromm

Mirror, mirror, on the wall, who's the fairest of them all?

The Queen

Am I ever going to get relief from this thing?

Dying Patient

In many ways, as pointed out in Chapter Four, the ruling idea of modern society is the idea of the self. While present day American individualism can be interpreted as a liberating force creating greater opportunities for individual expression, development and leverage, it needs to be remembered that the individualism of our age is not merely excessive but represents a movement away from commitment to the bonds of societal responsibility towards isolated and detached egoism [2, 3]. The widespread appeal of pop-psychology, with its gospel of self-affection, assertiveness, and personal fulfillment, emphasizes that the ultimate achievement of productive living is self-actualization and aggrandizement of the individual self.

Self-actualization, as Maslow envisioned it [4], did not nullify the value of shared human concerns and sociability as the contemporary thrust towards individuality does. Rather, in Maslow's design, the fulfillment of the "lower needs" for affection and self-respect necessarily takes place within a context of interconnection and mutual concerns. However, the quest for self-actualization in everyday American life largely nullifies the value of human interconnection and concern for others in preference to focusing energies on exalting the qualities of the self. In this sense, the ongoing American fascination with fame and celebrities is a useful indicator of our collective embracing of the value of self-exaltation.

An important dimension of the contemporary commitment to self is the American obsession with physicality. The ethos of "believing in me" has assumed a form that promotes a widespread attraction to diets, exercise, health consciousness, continuing commitment to the latest fashions, and an ongoing concern for presenting a physical image to others which is both attractive and admirable. The glorification of physical beauty is not a new phenomenon, or one that is uniquely American, but, as we soon shall see, the widespread societal commitment to physicality is a salient factor in stigmatizing dying people in the 1980s and 1990s.

Another major vehicle for satisfying the needs of the self is the pursuit and accumulation of material goods. Technological-capitalist society, as I discussed in the opening chapter, has socialized its citizenry to believe that commodity accumulation is an extension and reflection of self-worth. The American commitment to physical beauty and to materialistic consumption is also complemented by the growing American obsession with social and personal improvement: the honing of the skills and qualities that elicit a sense of admiration for the personal and social presence of the self. The development of personality skills, business techniques, and a sense of cultural sophistication have become important to the modern idea of self-satisfaction. Fromm takes this idea of the process of self-absorption to its logical extreme:

> Modern man has transformed himself into a commodity; he experiences his life energy as an investment with which he should make the highest profit, considering his position and the situation on the personality market. He is alienated from himself, from his fellow man and from nature. His main aim is profitable exchange of his skills, knowledge, and of himself, "his personality package," with others who are equally intent on a fair and profitable exchange [5, p. 88].

Like the Greek youth who looked into a pool of water and fell hopelessly in love with himself, Americans have established self-absorption as an eminent cultural value. The notions of self-expansion and beautification, pleasure seeking and fulfillment, grabbing for all the gusto, getting better all the time, and surrounding one's self with the finest things and the "finest people" are continually celebrated by American culture and its advertising media. When observing the contemporary American preoccupation with self and self-absorption, it becomes clear that the idea of the perfectibility of the self is an idea whose time has arrived.

IDENTITY PROBLEMS: BEYOND THE LOOKING-GLASS

As Fromm's citation which begins this chapter indicates, men and women are social beings. Our behaviors are distinct from those of our non-human animal counterparts in that they are largely defined and shaped by cultural and social forces. Not only is the formation of identity largely a social process, but the definition of the successes and triumphs, along with the failures and tragedies of the self, is in many important ways also a construct of social forces.

Charles Horton Cooley defines the dimensions of the self as factors that emerge from interaction and association with others. In his classic formulation of the looking-glass self [6], Cooley suggests that an individual is defined through one's own perceptions of another's evaluation of him or her. This is a process which has three principal elements: the imagination of our appearance to the other person, the imagination of the other's judgment of the qualities of ourself, and feeling and acting according to how one thinks others are judging these qualities.

The relevant point to be drawn from Cooley is that personal feelings of wellness or unwellness do not emanate from within an individual; rather they emerge from social interaction processes. Thus, within the framework delineated by Cooley, an identity problem is something that is associated with unsatisfactory feedback from others, or more precisely, one's perception of the disapproval of others. Orrin Klapp's well known study of identity crises characterizes an identity problem as any serious dissatisfaction with one's self: the feeling of being blemished, the feeling that "there is something wrong with me." [5]. These feelings of self-inadequacy are characterized by symptoms of self-hatred, being overly and excessively sensitive, time weighing heavily on one's hands, desiring to be someone else, and excessive concern over one's appearance [7]. Identity problems have emerged as a serious issue of study in the contemporary setting, as the existence of an identity problem represents a personal failure, that is to say, a violation of the goal of self-actualization.

While Klapp, Cooley, and traditional role theorists see the self in terms of face-to-face interaction with others, more recent scholarly efforts have indicated that the electronic media, particularly television, have been responsible for bringing images into the American home which shape and define the perceptions and identities of the viewing audience [8]. The electronic media, in their own unique way, have provided direct access to social information, social interaction, social values and social situations without requiring the direct presence of other people. In this way, television, through its particular means of communicating, interplays with human senses and perceptions in ways that influence individual definitions of social reality. The media clearly and strongly reinforce the values of individualism, materialism, physical beauty, and vitality. The media also forcefully promote images of success and desirability. Through the impact of their collective, representative images, the media identify personal qualities and traits that are culturally valued. To the degree to which the lives of television watchers are touched by this electronic medium and its messages, a foundation is laid for individual viewers to compare, contrast and evaluate themselves in relation to the standards which emanate from the screen. In this way, feelings of satisfaction, self-esteem, and success can be promoted in ways that do not require direct face-to-face interaction with others. Likewise, feelings of inadequacy, diminished self-esteem, and stigma can be promoted through an individual's negative evaluation of himself or herself in relation to the standards and qualities that flourish in the symbols and representations of the electronic media. In this way, a potential identity crisis can be spawned or exacerbated through the media.

The notion of a socially rooted identity problem is basic to understanding the human plight of dying people, but the concept does not go far enough to comprehensively explain the modern situation of dying patients. Consider the following illustration. A young obese woman who is fifty pounds overweight begins to feel dissatisfied with herself as she perceives signs of disapproval from others and as feelings of unhappiness with herself are fostered by the media. In an era of self-improvement, it is possible for this person to commit herself to a rigorous weight loss and exercise program in the pursuit of a new bodily self-image. If she achieves her goal, positive feedback from others and less dissatisfaction in her self-comparison to media images will mitigate her feelings of inadequacy. In relation to the problem of obesity, she is journeying toward a positive self-image free from many of the negative implications that are associated with the condition of being an overweight female.

It is important to recognize that many sources of dissatisfaction with one's self are potentially reversible. The conditions and causes of dying, however, are neither temporary nor reversible. Thus, while an application of the concept of identity problems is useful to study the predicament of dying people, its applicability is incomplete. The potential for transience and reversibility of socially-inspired sources of personal inadequacy make the concept of identity problems only partially and incompletely relevant for the study of dying.

The problems of dying are entrenched in the course of dying itself and the generalized devaluation of the dying experience by American culture. There is no culturally supported relief from these problems because the problems are fixed by and entrenched in the cultural definition of dying as a social evil. It is for this reason that a more stable and less temporal concept is necessary to portray effectively the horrors of dying for modern people. This is where the notion of escalator-social-stigma becomes a useful tool.

The term stigma refers to the disgrace of a person. It signifies something unusual, immoral, or bad about an individual [9, pp. 1-4]. Every society sets forth a range of qualities and behaviors which it prescribes as being desirable and an additional complex of attributes and behaviors which it proscribes as undesirable. Individuals who fall within the range of acceptable qualities and behaviors are said to be normal. Those who are ensconced in the range of undesirable activities and attributes are labelled as abnormal. In any given society those who, in the perception of the normals, are bad, dangerous or immoral will find that their identity is systematically tarnished and discredited. In this way, the existence of stigma represents not just a denigration of the different and deviant, but a defensive response by the collective normal citizenry to what is defined as threatening and tarnishing to their everyday lifestyle.

Goffman's theory on social stigma emphasizes that discrediting personal attributes are the essence of stigma. He describes how qualities discredited within a given cultural milieu lead to the stigmatization of personhood for any individual who possesses such qualities. Thus, as Goffman indicates, to be blind, crippled, mentally-ill, obese, or gay within American society is to be discredited by the world of the normals. A blind, gay, or crippled person in the operational framework of stigmatization is largely defined in terms of and through their discredited quality, the result of which promotes a generalized, stigmatized identity.

It is the presence of qualities of discreditability and the process of discrediting which distinguishes social stigma from an identity problem. A person who is shy, for example, may find it difficult to integrate easily into social gatherings and may feel blemished and inadequate as a result. However, in all likelihood, the consequences of the shyness could be contained and would not lead to the person's identity being publicly discredited. Thus, social stigma is a qualitatively more potent concept as it refers to those factors which disqualify and disengage a person from social acceptance and normalcy.

The strength of Goffman's thesis lies in his description and perceptive understanding of the injustices of social stigma. He correctly associates stigma with the devaluation of personhood and its corresponding feelings of anxiety, uncertainty and inadequacy. The weakness of his discussion lies in his failure to distinguish between the degree and extent of the social unacceptability of varying, and undesirable attributes. To be sure, some qualities carry greater potential for stigma than others. In addition, the degree and intensity with which a quality is discredited is naturally a significant factor which shapes the individual's reaction to and perception of his or her stigma. This qualification becomes especially important in relationship to the issue of death and dying.

In the literature on courtship and dating, Willard Waller discusses the processes involved in dating and how these processes lead to an escalation of intensity and commitment between partners. In his conceptualization, every step in the courtship process has a customary meaning and constitutes a powerful pressure toward taking the next step [10, pp. 727-734]. According to this principle of a continuing and progressive commitment toward greater intimacy, the couple is in fact journeying on a one-way-dating escalator. The more the escalator advances, the more difficult it becomes to reverse direction and escape the drift toward the final commitment: marriage.

The dying individual is also on an escalator. As critical disease progresses, physical well being regresses and the dying individual is swept along a downward path of pain, suffering, and deterioration. For all reasonable considerations, this downward journey is not reversible. Thus, unlike the obese person who can lose weight and look forward to a fat-free, positively reinforced future life, the dying person is irreversibly and totally encompassed by an unchangeable process. In this manner, the stigma of dying is a very special and unique stigma. In an age of self-actualization, perhaps it is not pressing too far to suggest that dying is the ultimate source of stigma.

Escalator-social-stigma, then, can be defined as the unilateral movement toward a totally encompassing, discredited state. Escalator-social-stigma is dying.

A salient exacerbating factor of the escalator journey of dying is an individual's negative evaluation of himself or herself—in isolation and/or in association with others. A revision of Cooley is useful here. His concept of looking-glass self implies an element of freedom in interpreting or imagining the perception of others. However, I am suggesting that the scope of this freedom is seriously restrained by the technological and narcissistic underpinnings of society. The increasing American emphasis on self and self-expression and the way in which the valuing of the self is grounded in the technocratic consciousness has already been established. As such, the social forces of individuality and a technological orientation become internalized by the American people, that is to· say, they penetrate beneath the surface of the skin and are infused into and become a part of the consciousness of the individual. As a consequence of a lifetime of continuing patterns of socialization, dying persons are likely to judge themselves as being inadequate—failures in light of the American value complex, and will draw strong, negative conclusions about their self-worth and the way others are perceiving them.

As the themes of hedonism, personal wellness, beauty, sexiness, and success are pounded home by society and its vehicles of communication, the narcissistic world view which is created will be influential in shaping the way we imagine others are judging and seeing us. Within this framework, dying persons facing the prospects of futurelessness, often feeling weak, looking thin and pale, and otherwise physically diminished, will be likely to make a negative assessment of their worth and other's judgment of them despite how others are actually responding and feeling. Coupled with the probability that significant others are acting in a confused and often helpless way, it is not difficult to envision the feelings of stigma that invade the dying person. It is in this way that the broader framework of technological society defines the parameters in which "looking-glass" assessments of the dying self take place. Thus, the forces of technocracy become dominant factors in discrediting the human identity of dying persons and in shaping their ultimate feelings of being blemished and inadequate.

THE STIGMA OF DYING: SCENARIOS OF PERSONAL TERROR

Dying people become discredited and stigmatized on the basis of a variety of dimensions that constitute the life experience of the dying process. A very common concern of the dying patient is: "I don't want my husband (or wife) to see me this way." This negative judgment about one's self and the perceptions of others is a highly normative factor of life for the dying patient, and reflects the base of inadequacy which shapes the self-perception of the terminally-ill patient. Pain, hopelessness, ugliness, anxiety and frustration are significantly associated with the modern dying scenario. The presence of these factors during the dying process wreaks havoc for the social and personal self of the dying individual.

Pain is a quality or experience that is without value to the modern definition of living. It is not difficult to see how many sectors of society conspire together to produce pain and its associated sufferings out of existence [11; 12, pp. 127-136]. When pain and suffering are not able to be controlled or contained, the individual is left to his or her private world of coping resources in dealing with the pain. The consequences of the absence of cultural systems of meaning and support during the presence of pain and suffering play a major role in shaping the everyday realities of dying cancer patients.[1] The world of pain and suffering, as described by dying patients themselves, convincingly makes the point:

> Pain, pain, pain . . . Sometimes it's so hard to describe the pain. It's a pain like . . . well, the way I feel when pain gets over me . . . It's like . . . EATING AWAY AT MY BONES.

Another patient, frustrated and increasingly disgruntled over the continued growth of his head tumor, comments:

> The pain is excruciating. It goes from my shoulder, up through my neck, and into my head, sometimes shooting right across my ears.

An additional patient adds:

> If you were to measure it on a scale of one to ten, the pain would measure fifteen. Simply a severe, severe back pain that inhibits mobility and inhibits appetite. With pain, you are not hungry. . . .
> The pain, it stops me from doing things I would normally do. Just moving is difficult enough, never mind raking leaves or going sailing. It's really the worst thing that can happen, the worst feeling that there is.

The typical sociomedical response to pain, from everyday life to the hospital into the hospice, is flight. Pain killers are regularly prescribed by physicians, aspirins are downed by the ton to alleviate hangovers, tension headaches and the like, and drug companies have been able to exploit the American intolerance of pain to very good financial advantage. Running away from pain, in a curious sense, has become a national pastime, unless in logical consistency with the American commitment to self-expression, the pain is something that is self-initiated, through an exercise regimen, for example. For the dying cancer patient, however, the pain is not self-originated and there often is little escape from the pain. Nor is there a justifying frame of reference or legitimizing slogan to provide purpose to pain. The idea of "No Pain—No Gain" is a slogan relevant to a particular

---

[1] Not every patient in my study suffered through the extremities of serious pain, but pain was a salient force in the dying experiences in that it *dominated* many of the life concerns of about half of all the patients in the study.

context of pain that is related to self-improvement and narcissism. It is wholly irrelevant in the life context of dying individuals. Pain thus is an uninvited, unwelcome, and ever present and haunting fact of the dying experience:

> The pain is always there. Even when it goes away, it's there. I know it will be back. I expect it.

Given the constancy of the pain experience, in a culture that devalues and avoids pain, it is only natural to expect that feelings of frustration and even hostility will arise in dying patients whose bodies are being ravaged by painful stimuli:

> When the pain starts, I wish I could get something to get rid of it right away. When I wake up and I'm not due for medication, I think: Oh God, what am I going to do?
> It makes me shaky and nervous. It's an incredible kind of tension. When I get that pain, I sometimes become angry and nasty. I get so desperate that I act in ways I shouldn't act. When I'm going through it, I just get so desperate.

The desperation that underlies the experience of pain results from two societal "failures." First, the forces of technology are failing the dying patient by their inability to successfully relieve "the worst feeling there is." During earlier phases of their lives, the gratification needs of many dying patients were well served by technology in that their comfort, luxury, and ideas of success were intimately linked with the pursuit and accumulation of material goods. Now, at a vital time in their lives, perhaps at a time when it has never been so desperately needed, technology fails to deliver on its promise to provide a transcendence of the human condition. In conjunction with the failure of technology, the American cultural complex fails the dying patient because it is unable to provide a blanket of support, solace, and meaning to the pain-ridden lives of dying individuals. It may be useful at this point to reflect back upon Ivan Illych's predicament and response to his culturally unmitigated pain and suffering experiences.

The unrelieved pain of dying often becomes so intense and severe that it utterly encompasses the life energies of the dying patient. As one patient observes, relieving pain and "again enjoying the pleasure of not being in pain" becomes the major driving force of the patient's life. Another expresses how salient the pain experience is to the world view of the terminal patient:

> Do you really think the pain will continue? That's all I'm really concerned about. Relief from the pain. . . .

Another patient comments:

> Going on and on for months and months in pain all of the time . . . that scares me. Deteriorating! Sometimes it gets so bad that I wish I could

> go just like that [snap of fingers] instead of suffering, and that's what you do with cancer. You just go down and down. Deteriorating, being in pain. Yes, that worries me very much.

Yet another speaks of the prime importance of the pain experience:

> I don't think I could tolerate the pain getting worse. If that comes, I don't know what I would do. If I had just one wish, it would be to be pain free. Yes, pain free. I'd be the happiest person in the world if I could get up and find myself without pain. Oh God, I don't know what I'd do. Go crazy . . . If that ever comes, oh God.

As depressing as it may sound, it needs to be recognized that the horrific nature of the pain of dying patients is logically understandable and even expectable within the cultural and social realities of technocratic society. This meaninglessness of the pain of dying becomes an additional source of stress with which the terminal patient must cope. One patient voices his dismay at the senselessness of it all:

> Purpose, meaning to the pain? No, no, no, no, no. I just keep asking myself: Oh my God, what did I do in my youth to be paid back with this kind of bullshit?

Another patient, in a painfully honest moment of reflection and insight, adds:

> The pain is evil. It's destructive, bad and even demonic. The cancer makes me nervous, anxious, obsessive. The pain and suffering is so bad that it must be evil.
>
> I often ask, what did I do to deserve this? I can't see any reason for pain. I can't see any reason for suffering. I can't see any reason, I really can't. If I had an explanation, it would set my mind at ease. Without it, there is just confusion; helplessness sometimes. I just can't be sure that there is a God. It's disturbing and uncomforting. Really, there is no meaning to the pain. Pain like this has to come from the devil. At certain times, I feel that the pain is punishing me. But for what? That I just can't see.

How vividly the fictional words of Tolstoy, on the meaninglessness of dying, leap to life. The four words: "There is no explanation!" may very well serve as the epitaph of dying in the twentieth century. In a society which values both the here and now of hedonism and the future orientation of success, it is not hard to see why the suffering and pain of dying is a feared and discredited human condition. Pain, by overwhelming the sensories with anguish and distress, violates the pleasure principles of social living and, as the above patient experiences indicate, becomes so pungent that it dominates the life experiences of the dying patient. In this way the metaphor of pain as an insidious evil, a meaningless monster to be conquered and avoided at all cost, becomes a reality for the lives of dying people.

In addition to and partially because of physical pain, the dying person is beleaguered by feelings of helplessness. A form of powerlessness, helplessness refers to the inability to accomplish the things that one expects one should normally be able to accomplish. It is characterized by feelings of impotence and insignificance, and may lead to feelings of worthlessness. As one patient summarized his dying life: "I really am no good at all."

The importance of individualism to the American way of life has been a central theme of my observations. It is this value of "moral individualism" which stresses that each person is his or her own keeper and responsible for his or her own self. Successful living is clearly defined on the basis of whether or not one is self-sufficient and capable of looking after one's significant others. The emphasis on defining the self in terms of detached individualism promotes socially based feelings of inadequacy (specifically helplessness) in the person who finds his or her ability to be independent and self-sufficient diminished and impaired.

Dying people regularly and freely speak about this burden of helplessness, of being unable to do the things they typically would do if they were not dying. One patient, in moderate to severe pain, contrasts her present predicament with lasting remembrances of the past. As she speaks, tears fill her eyes and flow down her cheeks:

> I used to be so active. I had a good youth. . . . Did so much and enjoyed life. I get to feeling so sad when I think about the things I used to do and how I can't do them anymore.

Another expresses the frustration of encroaching helplessness:

> I've had a good life. Now I'm shot though. This tumor . . . or cancer . . . or whatever . . . Well, let's just say I'm three-quarters shot. I just feel so sluggish. Oh, to have the appetite. To be able to do the things I used to do.

Longing to do the simple things normally done in everyday life and taken for granted by so many people blossoms into feelings of inadequacy as the downward escalator journey of dying progresses:

> I just hate this helplessness. The feeling of wasting away. I used to be able to do things for myself. To be able to take the train into the city and the subway up to the office for my treatment. That was good. Now, I'm so weak I can't even walk. I have trouble going to the bathroom without help. It's just all so scary.

Another patient tearfully voices her comments:

> I'm no good to anybody. Why am I living? Why doesn't God just let me die? I feel so useless, and I'm a burden to everyone. This is no way to live. The pain, oh why? I'm just no good.

Perhaps it does not take many words to capture the essential meaning of helplessness to the dying patient:

> I'm useless! I'm of absolutely no use to anyone.

The physical deterioration of the self with its accompanying diminishment of an individual's ability to live a normal life necessarily eventuates in an increasing dependency on others for the fulfillment of daily needs. This dependence often facilitates guilt when personal feelings of inadequacy are combined with the patient becoming a burden to others:

> I worry about my husband. He works, you know. And he comes to see me every evening. When I go home, he cares for me all the time. It's just not fair to him, for me to do this to him.

Another patient indicates:

> I feel guilty even when talking to my mother. She has enough to worry about without hearing all of my complaints.

This same patient voices her feelings about becoming a burden directly to her mother, after being informed by her doctor that there were no immediate plans for her release from the hospital:

> Mom, I want you to go home and take care of daddy. I'm going to be here for a long period of time, and I don't want you stuck with me.

The dilemma of the helplessness of dying patients becomes evident when we recognize that in an age of individuality one is subjected to increasing states of dependency on others. The predicament is further exacerbated by the detachment and alienation of our age which generates feelings of vulnerability among the dying, in that many of their emotional and social needs are inadequately met. A further complicating factor resides in the fact that the more the needs of the dying individual may be attended to, the more obligated and dependent upon others he or she becomes. This nullifies the ability to be self-sufficient and, in turn, fosters feelings of self-blame and guilt. In a curious way, the neglect of patient needs or the personal attending to the needs of the dying may in different ways both ultimately jeopardize the patient, resulting in an increase in his or her feelings of helplessness.

SEXUALITY AND DYING: FERTILE GROUND FOR STIGMA

Ideals of beauty and models of sexual attractiveness are extensively promoted in American society. Consider the following, not too facetious, description of the modern ideals of sexual physicality.

The "modern American woman" is a sexy being. Her slender stature allows for her firmly toned yet silky soft flesh to highlight her look. Her body may very well be at its best when tanned to an enticing brown. The fashion which adorns her generates mystery but hides nothing. Snug-fitting pants accentuate her lovely legs and shapely derriere. Her high heels alluringly add sensuality which is furthered by the properly seductive gloss of polish which graces her nails.

Her blouse is finely designed, loosely fitting but highly suggestive of the treasures that lie within. Her lips are red and full and add to the lustre and depth of her eyes. Her posture is one of independence; she's charming, vibrant, cultured and sensual. Indeed, the modern American woman has come a long way!? Where does one find this image being exalted? Not just in the expected sources of television, advertisements, films, and popular magazines, but also in such unlikely sources as *Ms*. magazine, whose advertising frequently and explicitly celebrates the virtues of the above-described ideal. I mention this not to denigrate the American feminist position, but to show how deeply and perhaps inescapably the ideals of feminine beauty are entrenched in our technological-narcissistic society.

The male counterpart to the modern American woman is differently but equally attractive. Tall, slightly muscular, well groomed, very handsome, and appropriately affluent, he too is a desirable commodity. His strength, intelligence, and success, combined with perhaps a newly developed modicum of sensitivity, create an ideal unparalleled in American society. Consider then, the erotic encounter which emerges when the American male and the American female unite in sexual interplay. Such a scenario would be so compelling that *Webster's* would offer its description as the primary definition of perfection.

These descriptions not only provide for a moment of diversion, but they illuminate the logical extreme of the American commitment to physicality, and they provide at least one image to which dying people compare their physical selves. It is at this point that the injustice of America's obsession with sexuality and ideals of physical attractiveness become apparent, namely, in the dehumanization, devaluing, and stigmatization of those who lack the qualities and necessary tools to fit into the prevailing definitions of sexy, attractive, and desirable. Indeed, it is not difficult to see how the obese, the disabled, the debilitated, and, of course, the dying are rejects of the American sexual model.

The more social and personal identity is defined in terms of sexual and physical well-being, the more the physical predicament of the terminally-ill becomes a source for stigma. Let us see how the physical implications of terminal illness affect the self-perception of patients:

> I used to be so happy. Really, I was a happy person and have been able and ready to go out and have fun. I've always felt good about myself and was always active socially and at home . . .
> I've always thought of myself as having a nice shape. Not being perfect, but having a nice body. Now, all of this has changed.

Another patient remarks:

> I used to be strong as a bull. I could hold my own with the toughest of them . . . don't you worry about that. But all I do now is lose weight. I'm not the same guy I used to be. I've lost so much weight that I don't even know myself. Look at me. I try to eat as much as I can. I love to eat, you know, but I don't have any taste anymore, and I get weaker and

weaker as I lose this weight. If I could only get stabilized. You know I used to weigh 220 pounds.[2]

A third patient speaks concisely of the impact of physical blemishment on her perceptions of self:

I'm not myself, anymore. Oh, the way I used to be. I can't even stand to look in the mirror anymore [tears begin to stream from her eyes].

Another patient expresses how her sexuality and self-concept have been tarnished and stigmatized by her radical mastectomy:

I don't feel the same way as I did before because of that breast not being there. I don't see myself being as sexy as before . . .

It's a big difference having one breast on one side and the other partially flat and scarred. To me, not having that breast there means that I'm not sexy anymore . . .

When I see other girls in low cut dresses or in a sexy bathing suit, I think to myself: Oh, I used to be like that, and I can't anymore.

Another patient expresses his feelings of sexual inadequacy and embarrassment over his colostomy:

As far as sex goes, I can't worry about that anymore. I just have to accept the fact that I can't do the things I used to do . . .

This goddamn bag though, is one thing that I can't stand. It smells, and it . . . ugh . . .

Well, what am I going to do if I'm at a dinner party, and it breaks? Then everybody would know, and that would be too embarrassing to take.

It is important to note that concerns about the stigma of the dying process and the blemishing of sexual-physicality, while of paramount importance to the patient, are dismissed as trivial and inappropriate by the medicalized world view of physicians. In fact, when the above colostomy patient made a similar complaint to his attending physician, the physician commented in a hallway conversation:

He's too much. He's worried about his bag breaking at a dinner party. Doesn't he realize that he's dying and won't be at any dinner party for the bag to break?

In another situation, a patient who had developed a secondary cancer site in her breast, was terrified by the removal of her breast and was expressing her fears and anxieties through asking an inordinate number of questions, many of which were repetitive, of her physicians. The patient became quickly labelled as inappropriate and a problem patient. Indeed, her surgeon upon returning from a post-operative examination and having totally nullified any consideration of

---

[2] The patient weighed 147 pounds at the time this statement was made.

the human side of her predicament, exclaimed to all present in the doctor's lounge:

> I don't see what she has to be angry about. She has a perfectly healed wound.

It may seem ironic in terms of America's obsession with sexual physicality that the sexual-stigma concerns of the dying patient are systematically ignored and denigrated. But, when considered in terms of the general devaluing of dying, the transformation of dying into a low status position in American society, and the attachment of a label of social death prior to biological death, it is not difficult to see why the human sexual concerns of dying patients are of minimal concern to the medical management of the dying process.

One of the major consequences of a diminished physical and sexual self-concept is the corresponding demise in adequate sexual functioning and the associated impact which this has on a patient's self-image. As one patient thoroughly describes:

> I feel very self-conscious about losing my hair. Really, I'm scared to start a relationship with anybody. I gained a lot of weight on my first chemotherapy, and that didn't help my image any. I felt lousy about my self-image and didn't like the way I looked . . .
>
> No, I'm not thin, mysterious, nor have gorgeous hair. Since the start of this cancer, I don't feel like a temptress at all. To think of myself as being pretty now, that's ridiculous. [She begins to laugh nervously.]
>
> I don't even feel a desire for sex, but I feel strange not having sex. I think you should have some kind of sexual drive, some kind of sex life. This I don't have, and it makes me feel inadequate and shy.
>
> This feeling of sexual inadequacy makes me avoid meeting people or beginning a relationship.

The same patient continues:

> I used to feel pretty confident . . . have a lot of confidence and be pretty outgoing. Now I feel shy and ugly . . . trying not to be noticed too much. I sort of withdraw and don't really like to go out too often.
>
> To a certain extent, I feel so much less adequate than before. I'm so very self-conscious. I feel like I don't know how to communicate anymore. You know, make conversation, small talk . . . So I avoid people very often.
>
> It seems that everything keeps going back to this cancer. It makes me feel so ugly, and it's just so depressing.

The ideals of sexual attractiveness which dying patients violate are often so deeply entrenched in the American psyche, especially among women, that even supportive outreaching from one's sexual partners and/or spouse cannot soften the consequences of physical and sexual stigma. The following patient benefitted from continuing support from her husband, whose genuine concern was for her

Watts School of Nursing Library
D.C.H.C.

well-being and recovery. Yet despite his warmth, acceptance, and love, her sexual stigma haunted their relationship:

> As far as sex life is concerned, we have been drawn apart . . . and all because of me. I know, I know, because of me.
>
> I feel funny. I just don't feel like myself, having that breast removed. I just don't feel 100 percent like myself.
>
> My husband told me it didn't matter. And I really believed him, but it was never the same. Me/myself felt different. Once again, we come back to that word "sexy."
>
> Although my husband continually told me that it was unimportant and that he loved me the way I am, I always felt that I am not good enough for him. That made me get out of sex by making excuses. I was always thinking about my missing breast.

The same patient continues:

> There was always something I was holding back. In my mind, I was always thinking: No, I'm not the same. Not the same. Even though he kept telling me it didn't make any difference. But to me, it's not the same.
>
> All the while I was making love, I would be thinking of how inadequate I was because of my missing breast. You better believe that this feeling made me want to avoid sexual relationships. I always had an excuse. I wasn't feeling well. . . .
>
> And after having made love, the feeling of not having that breast remained.

This is precisely the point where we find our revised version of the looking-glass self at work. Having internalized American values of narcissism and sexual physicality, it becomes difficult for physically blemished, dying people to imagine a positive presentation of self to others and to imagine that others are judging them favorably, even when others are doing exactly that. In this way, we find the technological-narcissistic strictures of our society unveiling themselves at the most personal levels of significance for the dying individual as feelings of sexual and personal inadequacy and stigma are an explicit consequence of the imprint of technological and narcissistic forces.

AS THE NEW SELF EMERGES

During the dying process, the dying person undergoes an identity transformation from a healthy, normal self to a new self beleaguered by debility and abnormalcy. The newly emerging self of a dying individual reflects the presence of many qualities that are disvalued and discredited by the complex of American cultural values. As one patient put it:

> If I could just go back to the way I was . . . used to be . . . then I'd be ready to die.

The negative self-image of the dying person entails both role transitions and the devolution of personhood. The self of the dying person is infused with a variety of discredited cultural traits on a permanent basis. This means not only that the self is torn apart but that dying irrevocably changes the roles that an individual will play for the remainder of his or her life.

One of the tragedies of modern living is that the role transitions of dying patients are not eased by cultural legitimations and support systems. As we have seen, the technical system of care is incapable of supporting the needs of the emerging self of the dying patient. The dying person, thus, is often left with a very private grief experience and is on his or her own in confronting the prospects of mortality. The resultant irony is that the individual is expected to engage (with dignity) the problems of dying through the use of personal resources, while at the same time he or she is trying to cope with the ravages of identity debasement and stigmatization. This is precisely what separates the evil of dying from other forms of stigmatized social deviance: *having to face the terrors of the ending of life while having the present torn away and blemished.*

The dying person is forced to fight a battle for meaning and legitimation without the necessary personal and social tools to wage such a war effectively. In this age of self-growth and expressiveness, however, some patients are able to successfully carve out a sense of purpose to their dying. I know this because it has been reported in the literature, but two points need to be emphasized in this regard. First, these successful attempts to engender a sense of tranquility and acceptance to dying are not reflective of culturally approved and institutionalized patterns of dying. To whatever degree individual deaths are relieved by heroic personal effort, hospices, and the dedication of "death-workers" such as Kübler-Ross, the private troubles of "X" numbers of dying patients are at least partially resolved. However, the public issue of dying, the ways in which the meaninglessness, stigma and neglect of the psychosocial needs of dying patients are rooted in the cultural and institutional arrangements of modern living, is never adequately addressed. In this regard, a salient method of organizing human death is the "psychologizing of death," namely, treating it as a predicament that is either resolved or unresolved on the level of private troubles. If dying with its attendant problems is successfully defined as a clinical-psychological management issue, society is freed from the encumbrance of having to establish and provide patterned responses to death and dying.

The second point is more simply put: there was not one patient in my study who expressed the feeling that his or her dying offered the possibility for creativity and growth. Indeed, every single patient consistently defined the prospects of dying as a regrettable and wholly negative force.

There are many patients who are not able to make the psychological adjustments that are necessary to cope effectively with their dying in positive and creative ways. Many of these patients employ a variety of psychically adaptive defense mechanisms to sustain them during the dying process. These include denial, avoidance of death-related conversation, living with the fight against terminal disease one day at a time, isolating themselves from ongoing social interaction, and the widespread use of metaphors to describe their battle with cancer. Despite many variations in trying to cope with the prospects of terminality, one image is consistently present in the lives of patients, namely, that of cancer as an enemy. One patient who was completely rational and appropriate until she was asked questions that touched the issues of cancer and death, illustrates how fearful patients can become of the enemy that is cancer/dying:

> There is this guy who is persecuting me. He comes into my house and takes my food. I had ziti in the refrigerator, covered with sauce and ricotta cheese, and he took off the sauce and the ricotta. He keeps taking my food. Tomatoes, which I also had. I guess the only way to get rid of him is to die. Everything new and nice which I have, he destroys. I can't have anything new and nice because of him. I have a nylon summer dress, and he shortened the length of it, and along the hemline, he made cuts. He cut it. I also washed and shined my kitchen floor, and he came and put black splotches all over it . . .
>
> He just destroys everything I have.

During another conversation, the same patient adds:

> He comes in during the middle of the night, and he steals everything I have. My pills [she was referring to the chemotherapy she was taking at home], he took them, one-half of them. I had a glass of water on my nightstand, and he took half of that.
>
> I can't keep food in the refrigerator, because he keeps stealing it. I've tried changing the locks, but that doesn't work. He picks the new locks, and once he does that, getting in is easy. I can't keep him out. I just don't know what to do.

Every time the patient was asked how she was feeling, the question would elicit a similar outpouring of bizarre metaphors such as these. Her interactional skills were normal in every other observable situation, and her doctors merely attributed her bizarre descriptions to her inability to face up to dying. Although it is beyond the scope of this work to delve into the psychological factors at work here, the fears and threats which this patient was feeling and coping with on a private basis are evident by her comments. It is especially interesting to note how "this guy" was taking away many of her life-sustaining forces: food, water, and medicine. Also, he either stole, shortened or blemished everything he touched.

In addition to psychologically rooted responses to dying, patients normatively place tremendous faith in the curative power of chemotherapy. Since comfort during the dying process is inhibited by many of the social factors already discussed, identification with the healing powers of technology provides some relief from the vulnerability and stigma of the dying process. One patient expresses her relief over the starting of a new regimen of chemotherapy:

> I'm so glad it's started. That he's back [referring to the attending physician who was on vacation] and decided to put me on medication. I was so afraid, and now things are going to be okay.

Another patient seeks to negotiate a bargain:

> Doctor, you remember the cars we talked about? The MG? Well, you cure me, and it's yours. I'm not kidding. If what you are doing works, it's yours.

The point to be made is that a myriad of coping mechanisms are employed by dying patients to support themselves throughout the dying process. These individualized patterns of adjustment, however, emanate from a self-image that is being seriously and permanently jeopardized by the downward escalator journey of dying. The dying person confronts and lives with a mixture of an ever-present gnawing anxiety and acute fear of dying and death. The pain, suffering, and helplessness of the low status, discreditable process of dying represents an acute and chronic endangerment of not just physical but also psychosocial well-being. This plight of dying human beings unfolds everyday in ways that touch deeply the lives of patients in hospitals all across America. Their plight is a real and continuing one, one which is too often hidden behind a veil of silence and avoidance.

Trapped in a diseased and protesting body and existing in a social order that has virtually no use for dying people, the dying person becomes threatened by a variety of external and internal forces. In many ways, dying people are the dregs of society. They are personally and socially insignificant, in that dying represents a progressively painstaking movement toward non-being or social death. In a nutshell, the external discrediting of dying in and by American society, along with internalized fears, anxieties and frustrations merge together in the making of a nonperson. The words of a dying patient best capture this stigmatizing force of the escalator ride of dying:

> Everything seems to lead me back to my cancer. Cancer, cancer, that's it! That's all there is. I'm just wasting my life away. There's absolutely nothing positive happening. It's [having cancer] all just so time consuming. It doesn't make me feel well . . . feel good or happy. It's boring and painful. Physically and emotionally, it's confusing and depressing. There's nothing positive! All it does is hurt. Everybody!

The words are self-expressive.

REFERENCES

1. E. Fromm, *Escape from Freedom*, Avon Books, New York, 1969.
2. R. Bellah et al., *Habits of the Heart*, University of California Press, Berkeley, 1985.
3. A. Etzioni, *An Immodest Agenda*, McGraw-Hill, New York, Chapters 2 and 3, 1983.
4. A. Maslow, *Toward a Psychology of Being*, Van Nostrand, New York, 1968.
5. E. Fromm, *The Art of Loving*, Harper and Row, New York, 1956.
6. C. H. Cooley, *Human Nature and the Social Order*, Scribner's, New York, 1922.

7. O. Klapp, *Collective Search for Identity*. Holt, Rinehart and Winston, New York, 1969, Chapter One.

8. J. Meyrowitz, No Sense of Place: *The Impact of Electronic Media on Social Behavior*, Oxford University Press, New York, 1985.

9. E. Goffman, *Stigma: Notes on the Management of Spoiled Identity*, Prentice-Hall, New Jersey, 1963.

10. W. Waller, The Rating and Dating Complex, *American Sociological Review*, Vol. 2, 1937, p. 727-734.

11. I. Illich, *Medical Nemesis*, Pantheon, New York, 1976, see especially Chapter Six.

12. D. W. Moller, On the Value of Suffering in the Shadow of Death, *Loss Grief and Care: A Journal of Professional Practice*, Vol. 1, 1986, pp. 127-136.

CHAPTER 7

Approaching Omega:
The Roller Coaster of Dying

Each society is a hero system which promises victory over evil and
death [1, p. 124].

Ernest Becker

The institutionalization of the dying patient effectively removes dying people
from the hub of everyday social intercourse and serves to help organize and contain the problems associated with the dying process. In many ways, the lives of
ordinary healthy people can proceed undisturbed by the terrorizing issue of
death, as the dying process is moored within a technocratic framework and isolated behind the total institutional walls of a hospital. However, hospital personnel often find their lives directly touched by death as the carrying out of their
professional role obligations requires interaction with dying patients. As we saw
in Chapter Three, varying medical respones to dying patients are linked together
through the medical profession's commitment to a technological orientation.
This technological coordination of human dying serves to submerge, "deny" and
organize the dying process into professionally manageable categories which restrain the expression of personal pinings about death and dying. As discussed in
Chapters One and Two, the idea of dying-with-dignity has been effectively
merged with technocratic strategies to create a broad societal base for the arrest
of potentially turbulent and disconcerting behaviors of the dying.

We have also seen how the values and priorities of the death-with-dignity
movement have affected the consciousness and behaviors of the profession of
medicine. In effect, many health care personnel have uncritically adopted the
credo of Elisabeth Kübler-Ross and have become travel agents for the dying.
Physicians, interns, residents, and even nurses often act to discourage expression
of the more hostile and emotionally charged "early stages of dying" and have
defined the proper role of dying patient behavior as facing up to dying with
courage and patience, i.e., dignity.

The unwillingness of medical professionals to accept dying patient behavior
which is publicly undignified is based on an assumption that dignity in dying
is possible and desirable. In addition, there is an underlying assumption that

83

predetermined, essentially linear, stages of dying exist. Consequently, if a patient is angry or difficult to interact with, he or she just needs to be transported to the acceptance stage. The purpose of this chapter is to examine the impact of technological management on the life course of the dying patient, paying particular attention to the idea of dying-with-dignity and harmonious adjustment of the dying patient's self to the terminal process. Before proceeding to this discussion, however, it is important to make some remarks regarding the concept of dying-with-dignity.

Dying-with-dignity has become an enormously utilized concept. There have been, however, despite widespread use of the phrase, few attempts to define or operationalize the concept. Dignity in dying, as it appears in the sociomedical, psychological and thanatology literature, refers to a non-specific, generic dying process. As one surveys the relevant literature, one finds the following themes frequently associated with the idea of death-with-dignity: courage; natural death; dying which is pain-controlled; tranquility; support systems; peace; spiritual meaning; and acceptance. There is, of course, no particular equation which defines the concept of dying-with-dignity. Rather, dying-with-dignity refers to an attitude and definition of dying that seeks to mitigate some of the undesirable aspects of medicalized dying. At the same time, dying-with-dignity seeks to recapture some of the sentiments and mores that are associated with traditional death patterns. In this way, dying-with-dignity is such a broad concept that it tends to become clinically useless. Nevertheless, it is useful in identifying a set of values regarding the meaning of human dying experiences and in unveiling societal reactions to technocratic death patterns. It is also important to note that dignity, as an overly general concept, has become part of the contemporary history, language and metaphors of dying. In both a general and specific sense, dying-with-dignity has become a significant frame of reference which defines part of the American cultural framework of death and dying.

When one looks carefully at the human realities of dying-with-dignity, two distinct types of dignity emerge. One has social meaning and prescribes for dying patients a restricted and inhibited course of behavioral and emotional expression. This type of death-with-dignity is related to the social organization of contemporary death patterns and leads to a therapeutically appropriate death process. The second type of dying-with-dignity has personal, existential meaning. This type of dying-with-dignity is related to the effectiveness of a person's private coping patterns and leads to an individually meaningful death process.

Personal dignity in dying is individually achieved. Therapeutic assistance, such as psychotherapy, participation in self-help groups or involvement in a hospice program, can contribute to an individual's personal achievement of dying-with-dignity. The individual, as we have already seen, is the primary basis of successful and unsuccessful personal coping with the fact of dying. Coping capacity, in this way, means far more than enduring physically the process of dying. It implies coping that has existential significance in terms of the search for meaning, the maintenance of personal morale, and coming to terms with death [2]. Achieving personal dignity in the course of dying may be, in Becker's theoretical framework, interpreted as a triumph over death. On the level of personal human existence, however, authenticity, purpose and meaning are its consequences. Coping well and achieving personal dignity may be one of the most dramatic existential statements an individual can make during his or her lifetime. Because physical survival alone has little significance for the human being, the pursuit of meaning becomes an essential challenge for humanity. If the quest for meaning is successful, of course that is good for the individual. If an individual succeeds in the quest for meaning at one of the darkest times of human life, the achievement is all the more inspiring.

Social dignity, unlike the existential significance of personal dignity, has purely interactional significance. One social dimension of dying-with-dignity emphasizes that dying patients should behaviorally respond to the process of dying with poise, restraint and even some courage. The significance of the social dimension of dying-with-dignity is that the process of human dying does not burden, disconcert or disrupt the activities of health care professionals who work with dying patients. The primary interactional significance of social dying-with-dignity is the facilitation of medical work for physicians and nurses. Dying patients achieve the social dimension of dying-with-dignity when they adapt their behavior and expressions to fit the requirements of the process of medicalized death. In this way, social dignity entails a therapeutically acceptable death process, which essentially means that a patient's behavior is acceptable within the framework of medical and technological management of the course of human dying.

In the social dimension of dignity there is little need or regard for personal dignity. Private feelings of dejection, disillusionment, despair, defeat, or even private suicidal inclinations are of little consequence to the management of dying patients. As long as correct patient behavior is maintained—as long as poise and courage do not give way to cantankerousness—the absence of private dying-with-dignity is of little concern to physicians. However, when private feelings of disillusionment, despair and anger are unleashed into the public arena, they become an issue for physician-patient interaction. The release and behavioral expression of private, negative feelings unleashes the issues of human dying. The personal dimension of dying-with-dignity becomes an issue for patient management when the private factors of a patient's inability to successfully cope with dying rage into the public arena and jeopardize the behavioral tranquility of social dying-with-dignity. In order to facilitate the technical management of the dying process, the private issues of non-coping must be sublimated to the social dimensions of dying-with-dignity. If this is accomplished, the once unleashed forces of human dying are again contained.

The distinction between private and social dying-with-dignity is essential to this chapter and the major themes of the book. The emphasis is clearly on the significance of social dignity in the course of technical molding of the dying process. The personal dimensions of dying-with-dignity become relevant to medical management only as they impinge upon the control of dying patients via the social dimensions of dying-with-dignity. This does not mean that the personal dimensions of dignity are wholly irrelevant. Clearly, they have relevance for the private, psychological lives of dying individuals, but that is beyond the scope of this study. Clearly, personal dimensions of dying-with-dignity are relevant inasmuch as they reflect the penetration of the human potential movement into the arena of human dying and death. Additionally, the personal dimensions of dignity are potentially relevant to the success of social dying-with-dignity. The degree to which dying patients are successful in achieving personal dignity in dying, their personal victory can be readily used as the foundation for establishing social dignity in their behavioral interactions with physicians. In this way, perhaps the ideal realization of social dignity is based on successful personal adjustment to the dying process. If personal success in coping with dying has not been achieved, various management strategies can be successfully employed to render "privately non-dignity patients" socially dignified in their dying.

THE COURSE OF DYING AND SOCIETAL FORCES

While Becker may be right in arguing that fear of death is a universal human trait, the ways which people seek to cope with the fears of mortality and seek comfort during the dying process are defined by the sociocultural sensibilities of the time and place in which they die. Historically, as I have already indicated, humanity lived in greater harmony with the idea of death, and the traditional deathbed was typically characterized by acceptance, fellowship and meaningful cultural rituals:

> Naturally [in the traditional pattern of death] the dying man feels sad about the loss of his life, the things he has possessed, and the people he has loved. But his regret never goes beyond a level of intensity that is very slight in terms of the emotional climate of this age . . .
> Thus, regret for life goes hand in hand with a simple acceptance of imminent death. It bespeaks a familiarity with death [3, p. 15].

As one chronicles the artistic and literary sources of traditional European and American societies, the theme of simple acceptance of death holds a paramount place. La Fontaine's portrait of the death of a peasant, for example, portrays the harmony that existed between human life and the process of dying. The dying peasant recognizes for himself that he is dying and gathers his children around his deathbed for final instructions and farewells:

> My dear children, he says, I am going to our fathers. Good-bye, promise me that you will live like brothers. He takes each one by the hand, and dies [3, p. 16].

As traced by the observations of Ariès and Stannard, the traditional orientation toward death began around the fifth century and lasted, despite variations in form, until the nineteenth century. The nineteenth century brought some changes in that it was an era whereby familiar simplicity was replaced by romantic, sentimental and overly inflated expressions of grief. It was also a time where fellowship at the deathbed was reduced from broad communal presence to a circle of intimate friends and relatives. Yet the peaceful sense of harmony between dying people and their process of dying remains a salient feature of the Victorian deathbed. Bram Stoker's novel, *Dracula*, classically portrays love and fellowship conflicting with evil and power, and offers scenes which memorably capture the harmony and intimacy of the deathbed. Lucy Westerna had been violated by Stoker's Prince of Darkness, and was lying on her deathbed, surrounded by a concerned and intimate circle of friends:

> For fully five minutes Van Helsing stood looking at her, with his face at its sternest. Then he turned to me and said calmly: "She is dying. It will not be long now . . . Wake that poor boy, and let him come and see the last; he trusts us, and we have promised him" [4, p. 168].

As Lucy's fiancé, Arthur, is awakened, the fellowship returns to her bedside:

> "Arthur! Oh, my love, I am so glad you have come!" He was stooping to kiss her, when Van Helsing motioned him back. "No," he whispered, "not yet! Hold her hand; it will comfort her more."
> So Arthur took her hand and knelt beside her, and she looked her best, with all the soft lines matching the angelic beauty of her eyes. Then gradually her eyes closed, and she sank to sleep. For a little bit her breast heaved softly and her breath came and went like a tired child's [4, p. 168].

As the scene progresses, Lucy again wakes:

> Very shortly after she opened her eyes in all their softness, and putting out her poor pale, thin hand, took Van Helsing's great brown one; drawing it to her, she kissed it. "My true friend," she said, in a faint voice, but with untellable pathos, "My true friend, and his! Oh, guard him, and give me peace!"
> "I swear it!" he said solemnly, kneeling beside her and holding up his hand, as one who registers an oath. Then he turned to Arthur, and said to him: "Come, my child, take her hand in yours, and kiss her on the forehead, and only once."
> Their eyes met instead of their lips; and so they parted.
> Lucy's eyes closed; and Van Helsing, who had been watching closely, took Arthur's arm, and drew him away.
> And then Lucy's breathing became stertorous again, and all at once it ceased.
> "It is all over," said Van Helsing. "She is dead" [4, p. 168].

The sensitivity of the foregoing passage is rooted in the mutually supportive interactions of the fellowship with the dying Lucy Westerna. Not only did the support of community participation in the dying rituals of the past provide for a sense of comfort and well-being to those who were dying, it was both a reflection of and partly a source of the simplicity and the harmonious acceptance of the coming of death. And as Stoker illustrates, even under the most extraordinary circumstances, dying was responded to as an ordinary and natural process.

As the twentieth century emerged, however, the images of tranquility and harmony that characterized traditional death were replaced by a new model of death: death as a social evil. As dying becomes shameful, ugly, and dirty, dying is perceived to be ordinary only under extraordinary circumstances. And, as we are about to see, the course of dying in a civilizational context that identifies dying as an evil to be denied or organized in the least disturbing way possible has become an uneven, turbid, and turbulent process. I am here not merely referring to the stigmatized horrors of dying depicted in previous chapters, but to the ambivalent and twisting course, the non-rhythmic integration of hope and despair, which is so much a consequence of the modern dying experience.

One of the inherent consequences of the medicalization of dying is the prolongation of the dying process. As disease progresses, medical-technological efforts to combat the disease and postpone death are intensified. In this way, the "natural progression" of disease is deterred by medical and surgical treatments which offer the dying person a sense of optimism and hope. However, during the course of terminal illness, improvements in physical states are often transient and temporary. This elicits a feeling of dejection and deflated hope as the disease and its symptoms progress. Of course, renewed medical efforts seek to moderate the progress and presence of the disease, and to the degree to which these efforts succeed, dejection is replaced by a rekindled flicker of hope. In this zigzagging process of dying, hope can be successfully used as a management mechanism to divert attention away from the disturbing and penetrating issues of dying and death.

Let us consider the emotional roller coaster ride of heightening hope and plummeting despair as illustrated by the following case study. A patient with a relatively unsuccessful medical history of lymphosarcoma was admitted into the hospital with severe swelling and pain in her abdomen. Her physician discusses some test results with her:

Doctor: The preliminary results of your CT scan show a growth of nodes, which are causing an obstruction. You have been urinating today— losing some weight—which is the first time you've done that since coming in. If that continues, we'll continue you on lasix to get the swelling down. If not, I'll ask Dr. ———— to radiate your belly [he points to the spot where radiation would occur] to see if we can't get the nodes to reduce. Then we can get you started on chemotherapy.

Patient: What will the medicine be?

Doctor: Some VMF, Methotrexate, some . . .

Patient: Could you write that down for me?

Doctor: When it comes time to start treatment, I'll go over the whole thing with you. Don't worry, you'll have plenty of advance warning.

Patient: For how long will I be getting the chemo?

Doctor: I'm not exactly sure what the protocol[1] calls for. I have to check it out. It'll be something I give you every three or four weeks.
Patient: Oh, so then we are talking about something overnight?
Doctor: Yes . . . , or I can give it to you in the office.

It is important to note how the patient selectively overlooked the initial concerns discussed by her physician and focused her attention on the specifics of her chemotherapy regimen, placing hope in the curative potential of the protocol drugs. The scenario resumes the following day after a physical examination and a review of specific symptoms and test results. The patient begins:

Patient: Doctor, so this isn't serious? [pointing to her severely swollen stomach]
Doctor: Serious?? [he hesitates] Well, your disease is serious. You do have extensive nodes [he points to her shoulder], and your swelling is probably due to node growth . . .
Patient: [interrupting] But it won't require surgery . . . ?
Doctor: No, that I can tell you for sure.
   . . . PAUSE . . .
Doctor: The critical thing is your swelling. We want to get that down with medication and/or radiation. That is the really important thing for now. Then we can begin to start you on some chemotherapy which will have a chance to work.
Patient: [focusing on the last phrase and showing visible relief] Okay, Doctor, good. That'll be fine. Thank you.

The patient is focusing on her hopes for the future. She is placing her faith in and relying on her expectations of the benefits to be derived from her anticipated chemotherapy treatments. She is, however, "naively unaware of how serious her condition is," as one doctor put it. Clearly, her doctors have been unsuccessful in communicating the nature of her diagnosis to her, and/or she has been selectively screening out indicators of bad news. In any event, this naiveté on the part of the patient was not very well understood by her attending doctors. Her primary oncologist, shaking his head in disbelief, commented to her radiologist in a hallway conversation: "She really thinks she is going to get well." And, the radiologist responded: "Do you mean she hasn't caught on?"

Chemotherapy had been discussed as a possibility with the patient. As a result of miscommunication between her attending physician, the house staff doctors, and herself, the patient had come to believe that the start of treatment was imminent. As it turned out, the intern and resident in charge of her case had wrongly informed the patient that she was to start on chemotherapy. The

---

[1]Protocol refers to a combination of drugs and/or procedures that have not yet been approved by the FDA for regular use but have been approved for use in experimental studies. The patient was being started on a protocol because she had already been placed on all the regularly prescribed regimens for her type of cancer, and each of those had ultimately proved ineffective.

attending physician, upon hearing this, reversed the order, citing two reasons. First of these was that his concern, at this stage of the patient's dying, was to make the patient feel as pain free and comfortable as possible. The interns aggressively argued with the attending physician on this point, emphasizing that they had an obligation to "try everything to save her." The physician was getting nowhere with the argument that treating her pain and other symptoms of discomfort was all that should be done. He then raised a second point, namely, that one of the requirements of the protocol was that the patient could not be edematous. Since the patient had severe abdominal swelling she was not, at this point, eligible for the protocol. It was this technical requirement of the protocol that prevailed upon the consciousness of the house staff doctors. At this point, they defined their professional obligations in terms of reducing the patient's swelling so active treatment could begin. Again, from the conflicting perspectives of the doctors involved in the care of this patient, we see how normlessness prevails regarding the ways in which patients should be technologically managed and in the definition of the ultimate goal of the medical management of the terminally-ill patient. Yet, we also see the centrality of technology to the divergent and conflicting forms of patient management.

The following conversation initiated at the request of the patient's parents, between the patient and a staff associate in the cancer center where she was being treated, illustrates that (for whatever the reason), the patient had not fully embraced the realities of her condition:

Patient: I'm just so relieved that they are going to start chemotherapy tonight.

Associate: You seem very enthusiastic about starting treatment.

Patient: Yes, [with a deep sigh of relief]. I just want to get better.

Associate: That is the hope of many people, but you should realize that being placed on the protocol does not mean an automatic, miracle cure.

Patient: What do you mean?

Associate: Dr. _____ told you of the seriousness of your condition two nights ago. Your disease is extensive, and he said it is spreading. It's important for you to recognize that the treatment will not make you well again, overnight.

Patient: It won't?!? [disbelief]

Associate: You've been on other combinations of medicine before, and you know that they work slowly, not rapidly. I hesitate even to discuss this with you, except that your doctors and I do not want you to be hooked onto expectations that are unrealistic and be shattered because of it.

Patient: Yeah.

Associate: If the treatment will have any positive effect, it will be only with you fighting along with it. The treatment will not instantaneously make you well.

Patient: Oh.

Associate: Have you thought about the seriousness of your condition at all?

Patient: No. I thought he said that I'd get well. . . .

The swelling in the patient's stomach was increasing and the attending physician decided to begin radiation treatment in order to reduce the nodes that were obstructing her kidneys, inhibiting the passing of fluids and causing her swelling. The early stages of radiation treatment brought some modest success. She was losing some fluid weight, but she was feeling increasingly weak and was in intense pain. At this point, as her swelling was being diminished, her doctors looked again toward the protocol. It was discovered however, that an additional requirement of the protocol was that the drugs could not be administered if radiation treatment had been received within the last thirty days. Her attending physician, recognizing that chemotherapy could not begin for at least a month, told the patient that he planned to finish up her radiation treatment and discharge her at the end of the week.

In recognizing that the hoped for and "promised" start of chemotherapy was not going to take place, the patient became increasingly depressed over the seriousness of her condition. A brief encounter with her mother expresses the re-emergence of a sense of despair and its superceding of the hope which had been previously alive and well:

Patient: I'm just so tired and feel so terrible.
Family
Member: But Dr. _____ said this wasn't serious.
Patient: I know I'm going to get better, but I just feel so lousy. Feeling this bad, I just don't know. I'm scared about this new protocol. That it may not work. I'm just so frightened.

The faith which previously had been placed in the new chemotherapy regimen had now been shaken, and the fear of not getting well became the dominant expressive and behavioral concern of the patient.

The patient was released from the hospital at the week's end, as there was nothing more medically that could be done for her. She was, however, readmitted several days later having difficulty breathing, visibly weak and in extensive discomfort and pain, and her abdominal swelling had again increased.

She was perceptibly nervous and disturbed by her worsened physical condition. This increased worry over her illness became explicitly expressed as an acute sense of fear:

> ... When will I be going home again? It's just taking so much longer than I thought. I just want to go home so bad. Do you think I'm even going to feel well again?
> I can't even describe the fear. There are no words ... It's too frightening for me to be able to describe. I'm just so afraid.

During the first two days of this readmission, it seemed that death was a likely possibility. Specific symptoms and key indicators were not encouraging. Her physician, at this point, was resigned to trying to make her as comfortable as possible and hoping for the best. Her fears during this period grew and her sense of despair heightened:

I'm afraid of dying. It really scares me. When I told you a month ago that I wasn't scared to die, I guess I was just denying it. Now I'm so anxious, nervous, depressed. I don't know how much more of this I can take.

On the third day of this admission her symptoms showed improvement. She had lost some fluid, her white blood count was up, creatinine clearance was improving, and her pain was easing a bit. She was generally feeling better, but it needs to be stressed that her cancer remained very widespread[2] and she was very, very sick . . .

Her physical symptoms continued to improve over the course of the next several days, and she and her physician seized upon these particular improvements. Her physician, who never even expected her to live this long, expresses his optimism over these improvements:

Doctor:	I think you are doing incredibly well. Your lungs and your belly have responded tremendously to the radiation we gave you. Certainly better than anyone ever expected you to.
Patient:	When am I ever going to start chemotherapy and go home?
Doctor:	We can't start chemotherapy until your creatinine clearance improves.
Patient:	Cre . . . ? Creatinine?
Doctor:	Creatinine is a waste product that is cleared by the kidneys into the blood. Right now, your kidneys are not operating sufficiently to clear creatinine as rapidly as should be. As soon as we correct that, we'll get you on chemotherapy.
Patient:	And that will help?
Doctor:	Oh, yes. It'll help you get rid of your lumps here and there [he gently points to the patient's kidneys and shoulder].
Patient:	These medicines work? You've used them before?
Doctor:	Yes, they are excellent medicines. No magic. They are just good medicines, and when used in combination, we hope to get beneficial results from them.
Patient:	When can I get started?
Doctor:	We want to get your belly flat first.
Patient:	I think it's flat now.
Doctor:	No, you've got another five pounds of fluid left, plus something over here [he probes her stomach]. We'll get that out, monitor the creatinine carefully, and then get you started.
Patient:	So by next Monday you'll be treating me?
Doctor:	I hope so.[3]
Patient:	Okay, Doctor. Thank you. Thank you very much.
Doctor:	[preparing to leave] You're doing incredibly well. Your lumps in your belly are rapidly diminishing. Your legs are doing well,

[2] She had obvious and visible growths of tumor on her forehead, around her armpit area, and on her vagina, in addition to the internal growth of nodes.

[3] The patient had become so sick that the attending physician, with full support of the house staff physicians, was considering giving her a chemotherapy treatment despite her having been radiated within the past thirty days.

and your belly has been really flattened by the radiotherapy. You are doing spectacularly. Again, far better than anyone thought you would.

At this point the despair, which the patient brought to the hospital and felt deeply early on during her readmission, has been replaced by a rekindling and stirring of the fires of hope. The patient, however, died three weeks later, never having been placed on the much-hoped-for chemotherapy regimen. Her attending physician was on vacation at the time. . . . It is almost staggering how abruptly the lingering, roller coaster journey of dying can come to a halt.

The emotional roller coaster journey of the patient from hope to despair back to hope again . . . is largely a consequence of peaks and valleys ·in the progression of physical disease and the patient's perception of the disease. Both of these phenomena are, however, largely the consequence of the modern approach to dying, namely, "denial" and technical intervention and management.

Hope is the last refuge from total psychosocial annihilation from the horrors of modern dying. Through technical intervention, a variety of specific symptoms can be treated and ameliorated during the dying months, weeks, and days. By concentrating attention on particular symptomatic improvements, the physician is able to avoid confronting the distasteful issue of a patient's dying. Converging attention on improving symptoms also offers patients a haven of hope through facilitating a world view that is subjectively more optimistic than could be legitimately defined from their objective disease state. When the disease progresses and symptoms correspondingly worsen, physicians can still comfortably dodge the issue of dying and death by isolating their attention on the exacerbation of disease-symptoms and their treatment. The patient, however, cannot remain on such an even keel as the worsening of symptoms clouds hope and injects despair and pessimism into the patient's definition of his or her future.

The roller coaster journey of dying is a pilgrimage defined by the management of dying patients through technology. It is distinctive from the ritual and fellowship which promoted a sense of harmony between the dying person and his or her own mortality during the eras of the tame and traditional ways of death. It is important to note that the roller coaster of dying, as generated by the medical manipulation of the symptoms of the dying process, is functional for the medical staff and the hospital system. In this framework, a physician can restrict his or her attention and activities to biomedical intervention into the disease process and can divert attention away from the haunting question of living versus dying, to the more manageable issue of the treatment of fragmented bodily parts and processes. If a physician were unable to find a way to define and organize dying within a technological framework, he or she would be regularly exposed to the personal, human forces of the dying experience. As we have already seen, physicians do not desire and are ill-prepared to confront the personal, psychological and social facts of human dying.

The technical molding of the dying process, with the sharp twists and turns of the roller coaster, serves to maintain the dying patient within the strictures of the sick role. This focuses physician and patient energy and attention on specific bodily parts or physical symptoms. The result sets the stage for the dying patient to be treated within the institutionalized expectations and corresponding set of sentiments and sanctions [5, p. 436], that are applied to any other medical patient. According to Parsons' well known formulation, the deviancy of illness is legitimized through the creation of the sick role. A person becomes excused for one's illness, that is to say, illness is legitimated and made socially acceptable, as long as the individual adheres to societal expectations set forth for him while he or she is sick [5, pp. 436-437]. These behavioral, definitional role expectations have four major dimensions. The sick person is not responsible for the illness condition and hence must be cared for. In addition, the sick person is exempted from normal social responsibilities; work, school, etc. The third dimension of the sick role is the obligation placed on the person to want to get well. The final requirement is that the sick person seek competent professional-medical help and cooperate with that help in order to be well again.

The traditional use of the sick role is based on the assumption that the condition is not permanent. Hence, dying or more precisely the dying patient, would not seem to be legitimately included within its parameters. The discussion of the downward escalator journey of the dying patient indicated how dying progresses without realistic opportunity for reversal. However, as indicated in this chapter, the (unchangeable) course of dying is often ignored by physicians and patients as specific symptoms and the medical treatment thereof become the center of the doctor-patient interaction. In the degree to which this occurs, the dying person is treated like any other patient and the sick role becomes an "illegitimately legitimate" category for classifying the dying patient. It is illegitimate because of the diversion of attention from dying to the management of symptoms, and the corresponding illusion of optimism which is created, the combination of which, allows for the sick role to become relevant to the management of the dying patient. Since the physician is narrowly focusing attention on the specific physical conditions and the patient does tend to focus on these as indicators of generalized improvement of health-disease status, the dying experience is frequently framed by normative expectations of the sick role. Thus, in a curious way, because of technical intervention, a technocratic definition of reality and the resulting roller coaster ride, dying patients and doctors relate to each other through the specificity of sick role performances.

'Peaks of well-being' during the dying process are largely doctor defined and technically induced. Thus, the technological organization of dying adds periods of peaks and valleys to the generalized downward trodding of the escalator path of dying. This up and down movement between hope and despair is not at variance with escalator dying, but rather is one variable form of the process of physical, emotional, and social deterioration, which is dying. In a sense, the climb toward renewed hope does not necessarily divert the escalator from its downward journey but rather serves to delude the patient about where he or she is journeying, thereby creating false hopes and unrealistic expectations. The information that "today your symptoms are not doing well" deflates hope and brings concerns about death to the fore. Tomorrow's message that "your symptoms are doing better; are doing well" reinstates hope and relegates concern about dying to the private backstages of human consciousness. In this way, the dying process in American society is characterized by the turbulence of technical manipulations of physical symptoms and changing patient hopes or expectations for the future. It is precisely this turmoil and turbulence which is a characteristic part of the downward escalator movement of the dying process.

As the sick role is cast upon dying people, patients are socialized by the medical staff and their associated role expectations to focus their attention on the treatment of specific, often isolated, physical symptoms. In this way, the emphasis on physical symptomatology not only encourages unrealistic patient expectations, but functions to restrain patient emotional expressions related to the stigma of the dying experience. The imposition of the sick role becomes then an effective vehicle for controlling the disturbing and distasteful psychosocial outpourings of dying patients. Of course, this is of use to the physicians and the hospital system as the flow of medical work is not stymied by emotional turbulence.

The ambivalence and the emotional jockeying of the roller coaster of dying not only diverts attention away from considerations of death and dying but also individualizes the grieving process. Focusing attention on physical symptoms, and doctors defining the treatment of disease and its symptoms as the only real concern of their professional role expectations and obligations, means that frontstage expressions of grief will be negatively sanctioned by medical professionals. Thus, the roller coaster, sick role treatment of dying patients, while not able to eliminate anticipatory grief from the terminal process, facilitates the privatization of grief, as expressions of emotion related directly to dying are defined as an inappropriate component of the technological management of death.

In addition to helping to assure that grief does not spill forth into the public realm of doctor-patient interaction, the stress upon treatment of symptoms and the application of the sick role to dying patients serves to de-emphasize the specialness or uniqueness of dying. Dying, in this way, is transformed into something ordinary and, as dying becomes ordinary, it becomes organized into the thread of everyday life in ways that are neither dramatic nor disturbing. Making death, which is alien and threatening to modern sensitivities, ordinary serves to ensconce the process of dying neatly into the everyday, standardized, bureaucratic routine of the hospital. Thus, dying is stripped of the public expression of many of its disturbing and perturbing factors. In this way, the horror of dying and the rage of dying patients are contained or, to borrow from the language of Ariès, death itself is tamed.

In short, the windfall of ambivalence created by the roller coaster of dying is one form and consequence of doctors dancing around the truth-of-the-truth; of avoiding the harsh sociohuman realities of dying. As we have seen in this chapter, there are at least two ways of not thinking about death: the way of our technological civilization which finds ways of refusing to talk openly and honestly about death and, the way of traditional civilizations, which is not so much a denial of death but a recognization of the impossibility of dwelling on death for very long and hence emphasizing the comforting roles of fellowship, ritual, and ceremony. The roller coaster of dying, with its emphasis on the applicability of the sick role to the dying patient, is a manifestation of the American attempt to organize and control human death. It is a means of encouraging silence, social dignity, and even some optimism on the part of the dying patient which, in effect, become practical mechanisms of death management and dying 'denial.'

REFERENCES

1. E. Becker, *Escape from Evil*. The Free Press, New York, 1975.
2. A. Weisman, *The Coping Capacity: On the Nature of Being Mortal*, Human Sciences Press, New York, 1986.
3. P. Ariès, *The Hour of Our Death*, Alfred Knopf, New York, 1981.
4. B. Stoker, *Dracula*, Ballantine Books, New York, 1959.
5. T. Parsons, *The Social System*, The Free Press, New York, 1964.

CHAPTER 8

A Concluding Statement on Technology and the Social Isolation of Dying

The old man closed his eyes. As life carried away the rumblings of the town, and the heavens smiled their foolish, indifferent smile, he was alone, forsaken, naked, already dead [1, p. 26].

Albert Camus

There is a notable tendency, on the wards of medical centers and in the broader society in general, to isolate human dying and death from the mainstream of human activity. Dying is excluded from social life through the isolation of children from death, by the absence of traditionally grounded social rituals to guide dying people, and by the growing expectation that dying and death are experiences that should properly remain within the confines of an individual's private existence. Dying is excluded from the medical world, in that dying is normatively transfigured into a chronic-illness state which elicits symptomatic palliation in treatment, and provides a framework for isolation of the "big" question of a patient's dying from the more narrowly focused, technical issue of symptom management. In this way, the human issue of dying is isolated and excluded from the bulwark of medical-technical activity, i.e., from the standard-ized routine and orientation of medical work.

The American faith in science and technology and the shared cultural com-mitment to individualism are seminal forces which underlie the social isolation of dying in America. As discussed in Chapters One and Two, technocratic-individualism generates a frame of reference for everyday social living which is in contradiction to the realities of the human experience of dying. The images of death which abound in our society, the ideas of dying and death which typify our age, and the behavioral manifestations of those images and ideas are salient sources of socialization about dying and death. It is within this frame-work that dying is isolated from the positively esteemed, sought after values and meaningful experiences in American society. Of course, this process of socializa-tion and subsequent internalization of attitudes and images regarding dying and death, becomes part of the character-personality structure which defines an indi-vidual person's relationship to dying. Specifically, not only are ideas and images about dying and death culture-bound, but as these images become instruments of socialization, they function to influence an individual's perception of his or her own dying and facilitate or inhibit the ability of the dying person and surrounding community to adjust to the experience of dying.

As images of dying and death arise in a specific cultural and historical context, the medicalization of death has emerged as a structural reflection of the specific cultural images and circumstances of contemporary American society. The medicalization of death thereby is not only reflective of the dominant images of dying and death in the technocratic social setting, but is one vehicle by which the prevailing images of death and dying become translated into observable social realities. Specifically, the idea of death as a social, community, and natural process becomes redefined into a scientifically manageable and preventable phenomenon:

> More than ever before, we can hope today, by the skill of doctors, by diet and by medicaments, to postpone death. Never before in the history of humanity have more-or-less scientific methods of prolonging life been discussed so incessantly throughout the whole breadth of society as in our day. The dream of the elixir of life and of the fountain of youth is very ancient. But it is only in our day that it has taken on scientific, or pseudo-scientific, form. The knowledge that death is inevitable is overlaid by the endeavor to postpone it more and more with the aid of medicine and insurance, and by the hope that this might succeed [2, p. 47].

When one thinks of a person dying in modern civilization, hospitals, machinery, drugs, professional staff, alienation and a sterile environment typically and readily come to mind. In a way, these ecological realities of the dying patient's contemporary environment have become standardized symbols reflecting the peculiarities of medicalized dying. The salient point to be emphasized in regard to medicalization of dying, as a reflector of and contributor to prevailing images of death in the broader technocratic society, is that medicalization of the human dying process isolates dying patients from their own dying experience. The medical education of student doctors, the professional activity and norms of medical work along with the technologically based orientation of the profession, all function to disengage dying, as a human experience, from the professional frame of reference which defines the course of physician activity. Of course, as seen earlier, there are a variety of means by which physicians transform dying into a medicalized phenomenon. Closed-awareness contexts where truth is hidden, obscured, or sugar-coated are very much in full use as a means of isolating dying and its experiences from the mainstream of physician-patient interaction. The technologically based, save-at-all-costs orientation, as well as the avoidance-neglect and sympathetic-detachment orientations, are additional ways in which physicians isolate dying from their arena of professional activity. Consequently, the patients' experience of dying becomes excluded from the array of interactions with their doctors.

The variability of physicians' attitudes regarding how "dying patients" should be managed, the lack of norms to guide physicians in their interactions and communications with the dying, and the general fact that physicians tend to relate to the dying patients in ways which doctors find most personally easy and comfortable, further contribute to the isolation of dying in the medicalized framework. Dying is excluded from the shared professional culture of physicians and, to the extent that physicians are the umpires and arbitrators of medicalized death, dying is also excluded from the realm of appropriate content for patient interaction with physicians and vice versa.

In addition to dying being isolated from the interactional world of doctors and patients, the bureaucratic organization of the modern medical center excludes many of the human needs and experiences of the process of dying from its fairly standardized definition of appropriate professional-organizational activity. Indeed, the values of affective-neutrality, efficiency, detachment and rationality—which preeminently underlie the operation of the modern medical center—are not conducive to the presence of any tasks, concerns, and issues which threaten to disrupt the standardized and efficient, medical work routine. In this way, from the viewpoint of institutional expectations, the dynamic, emotional state of human dying is neutralized by the bureaucratic organization of modern medical care. The affective state of dying is thereby excluded from the operational mainstream of bureaucratic medical activity. In this sense, dying is relegated to and contained in the individual patient's private or personal frame of reference. Thus, the human experiences of dying are pushed farther and farther behind the scenes of medical work and isolated from the public arena of medical activity.

A dominant tendency of the broader technocratic society is the drift away from community and moral solidarity toward isolated individualism. Themes of moral estrangement, spiritual isolation, and interpersonal fragmentation pervade contemporary society and the scholarly study thereof. In Nisbet's perceptive words:

> To examine the whole literature of lament of our time—in the social sciences, moral philosophy, theology, the novel, the theatre—and to observe the frantic efforts of millions of individuals to find some kind of security of mind is to open our eyes to the perplexities and frustrations that have emerged from the widening gulf between the individual and those social relationships within which goals and purposes take on meaning. The sense of cultural disintegration is but the obverse side of the sense of individual isolation [3, pp. 9-10].

The historical sense of community, which flourished in predeveloped Western Society, has been extensively discussed in the academic literature. For our purposes here, two major points are salient. First, traditional ties of community bound individuals together in a framework of moral imperatives, social rituals, and social stability. Second, in specific relationship to death and dying, community presence and traditional rituals of dying facilitated, or perhaps it would be more correct to say mandated, that dying be a culturally shared community experience. Thus, dying took place not just in the public presence of community but within a frame of reference that was characterized by standardized behaviors, common assumptions and shared cultural meanings.

As Western society developed economically, industrially and politically, community and tradition began to lose their base of authority. Two major points are again relevant. First, the moral certainty which is a by-product of communal living has been replaced by secular individualism, the result of which is that quests for meaning are increasingly divorced from a shared communal base and are more and more pursued by individuals independently of each other. The insecurities, moral dilemmas, and normlessness which typify our age, not only reflect the absence of shared cultural meanings and norms, but are situations which increasingly confront the individual in personal ways. Individuals must respond to these situations on the basis of their personal resources and abilities. Second, in relation to death and dying, the human experience of dying has become isolated from shared, communal meanings. The result is that the meanings of dying are increasingly privatized and individualized. The absence of shared cultural norms and the individuation of meanings of dying serve to isolate the dying patient, his or her family, and friends from each other into private, encapsulated worlds of survival and coping. This increases alienation of the dying patient, as it also exacerbates the instabilities and normlessness of the dying experience by separating the participants into privatized spheres of meaning and coping.

The escalator-social-stigma of the dying process is a lamentable outcome of the social isolation of death in American society. In a most fundamental way, the dying patient is isolated from those qualities which are valued in American culture, from those which provide a seedbed for self-esteem and self-affirmation, as well as those qualities which provide a base for interconnections and interactions with others. The pain and suffering that often typify the experience of dying are unmitigated by cultural legitimation. On a most basic level, there is no legitimizing motto or motif for the pain of the dying process. The American idea of "No Pain—No Gain" becomes null and void in the circumstance of dying and death. In the absence of a culturally grounded meaning system for suffering and pain, pain and suffering have become defined as clinical issues requiring therapeutic, medical management. In this way, the pain of dying is isolated from the web of social and cultural systems of meaning. I do not mean to overromanticize the role that culturally moored support systems played for dying people in traditional, Western society. Unquestionably, in an age of death from infectious disease and pestilence, many people died very painful and agonizing deaths. Clearly, medical technology has achieved some significant results in controlling and managing the physical agony of the dying process. Yet, even in this age of hi-tech medicine, physical pain remains a salient—and very much feared—dimension of dying. But as the response to the pain of dying has passed from the hands of family, community, and social or religious rituals to medical technicians, when the limitations of biomedicine in controlling pain prevail, the dying patient is left to face his or her pain and associated suffering in an isolated and privatized world of coping and endurance. In this way, while the technological management of the pain and suffering of dying has positively contributed to reducing some of the physical agony of dying, it has simultaneously resulted in a heightening of emotional and social isolation of the dying patient.

The emotional, cultural, and social isolation of the dying patient from the community of the "well and living" is associated with the loss of self-esteem, identity deterioration and blemishment. In our age of individualism, with increased value placed on self-development and expression, dying is the ultimate decimator of the American pursuit of narcissism. Helplessness, vulnerability, despair, physical devolution, and sexual blemishment impact the dying patient in such a devastating way that the social stigma of dying isolates dying patients from the community of the living, facilitating social death before biological death. The scenarios of personal terror recounted in Chapter Six illustrate not just the identity diminishment of the dying patient but also highlight his or her personal and social impotence. Traditional social rituals of dying, in a straightforward Durkheimian sense, provided a common base of participation and a sense of belonging. These rituals served to attach the dying person to the community of the living. In addition to generating a sense of group cohesiveness in the face of dying, traditional social rituals facilitated a sense of strength and transcendence, as the dying person became thickly attached to the moral order of the surrounding community. Also, it should be remembered that the traditional social rituals of death were both reaffirming of and reaffirmed by prevailing cultural values. In this way, the dying person was integrated into a cultural framework of meaning that provided for moral and social significance for the dying person.

The absence of rituals, institutionalized interconnections with the community of the living, and the lack of culturally sanctioned meanings to dying leave the dying patient morally, socially and personally insignificant. This really is the underlying basis of the escalator-social-stigma of dying, namely, the fact that personal and social death precedes biological death. Thus, the problem of meaninglessness asserts itself, for dying patients, not just in an abstract, existential way, but in ways that have concrete, deleterious effects for the personal and social identity of dying individuals.

The fact of death is in the nature of being human. More significantly, however, it is in the nature of humanity to be aware of the fact of mortality and to seek some means of coping with the inescapable fact of death. Indeed, since the beginning of the human race, human beings have had to come to terms with or find some means of adjusting to death. In American society today, the dominant means of adjusting to death are the technological management of dying and the growing expectation that one should die a socially or personally dignified death. Social dying with dignity minimally means that one should not publicly distress others by one's dying. Maximally, dignified death means dying in a way that transforms the dying process into a final opportunity for self-enhancement, growth, and an individually inspired quest for meaning. While the model of technological management is the dominant means of controlling the dying process and facilitating social dignity, the idea of death-with-dignity has gained widespread recognition and, as I have already discussed, is very much consistent with both the narcissistic and the technological underpinnings of American society.

As death in American society has become divorced from rituals and culturally legitimized systems of meaning and is increasingly characterized by meaninglessness, terror, devolution, normlessness, and stigma, new forms of controlling and managing dying and death have necessarily emerged. Modern management through death-with-dignity and through technological manipulation of the dying process is a way of suppressing and containing the tribulations of dying in a fashion that minimally disturbs and threatens the world of the living. And in different ways, the social and personal dying-with-dignity mandate and technological management facilitate the social isolation of the dying patient.

Personal dying-with-dignity places the burden of successful and appropriate death squarely on the shoulders of the individual. In this way, good death is isolated from collectively shared social codes, norms, and rituals, and the quest for dying a good death leads the dying patient away from commonly based systems of meaning and toward private and isolated definitions of meaning. But, as I suggested earlier, it is also largely unrealistic in a society which excludes dying, suffering and death from the course of everyday activity to expect that individuals will be able to successfully make the social and psychological adjustments that are required for death-with-dignity. In this way, a lifetime of socialization for successful living in a narcissistic, technocratic social setting precludes and excludes the dying patient from a dignified and meaningful dying experience. (This does not mean to assert that some individuals cannot heroically achieve a dignified death but rather refers to normative societal patterns of dying.) There is no doubt that the patients in this study found personal dying-with-dignity to be unrealistic and problematic for their lives.

Redefining the process of dying into the contours of the sick role, together with the subsequent roller coaster journey of hope and despair, serve to exclude dying from the dominant frame of reference of the dying patient. The technological management of death is an important means of managing dying in the modern medical setting and of facilitating social dignity. In this way, technology has replaced tradition and ritual as the prevailing defense against death and dying. But, as the community of the living becomes less and less involved in the process of dying, not only is dying stigmatized and culturally denigrated, the psychological and social agony of dying individuals is exacerbated. In an age where medicalized death has achieved an unparalleled sense of sterility, hygiene and perhaps even physical comfort, an emotional, personal, and social turbulence has simultaneously been unleashed. The turbulence that rages with respect to dying is responded to in isolation, through therapeutic and technological management of the individual patient's path of dying. The isolation that dying patients may feel is so total that their suffering, fears, and even their very lives, become increasingly invisible in a social setting where people have other things on their minds than suffering, dying, and death. This, perhaps, is the ultimate irony of modern civilization, namely, that in an era where the value of the individual has never been greater, the value of a dying person has never been more diminished. In an era where technology has contributed greatly to the diminishment of human pain and misery, the suffering and agony of isolated dying rages unmitigated. The despair of the dying patient, caught in the levels of complexities of the modern social setting, is obvious throughout this book. Now, it is up to you, the reader, to decide if we as a society are justified in despairing as well.

REFERENCES

1. A. Camus, Irony, in *Lyrical and Critical Essays*. P. Thody (ed.), Vintage, New York, 1970.
2. N. Elias, *The Loneliness of the Dying*, Basil Blackwell, New York, 1985.
3. R. Nisbet, *The Quest for Community*, Oxford University Press, New York, 1953.

A Methodological Note

... sociology is an inherently controversial endeavor [1, p. 3].
Anthony Giddens

The social and cultural landscape is as much the province of the sociologist—or novelist or poet—as the physical setting is of the painter [2, p. 43].
Robert Nisbet

Fieldwork, then, provides a mirror for looking at who we are as over and against who we would like to be. It provides us with soft data-observations, intuitions, and comments—for rethinking some very hard questions about what it means to be a member of the society [3, p. 14].
Charles Bosk

One of the hallmarks of the sociological tradition is the penetration of official and orthodox explanations of social living. The discovery of non-obvious systems of meaning and insight that go beyond the smokescreen of official rhetoric, and the unveiling of patterns of human living that are obscured or hidden by the cultural and social arrangements of society, are of central importance to the mission of sociology. In this way, as Berger aptly describes, sociology fulfills an important debunking function:

> We would contend, then, that there is a debunking motif inherent in sociological consciousness. The sociologist will be driven time and again, by the very logic of his discipline, to debunk the social systems he is studying ... The sociological frame of reference, with its built-in procedure of looking for levels of reality other than those given in the official interpretations of society, carries with it a logical imperative to unmask the pretensions and the propaganda by which men cloak their actions with each other. This unmasking imperative is one of the characteristics of sociology particularly at home in the temper of the modern era ... [4, p. 38].

Clearly, the debunking motif of sociology entails not just searching for unadmitted and hidden aspects of social life. This approach also carries with it a responsibility to confront and study unpleasant and unappealing aspects of social living. In this way, not only does sociology seek to debunk the hidden and taken-for-granted interpretations of social living, but it nurtures the development of a critical sensitivity in the exploration of salient issues that affect the condition of human life, especially in the modern societal context.

This critical sensitivity is at the core of what C. Wright Mills termed the sociological imagination [5]. In adopting the style of sociology which Mills advocated, I have sought in this book to explore dying as a public issue, defined in terms of the cultural and social facts of modern American society. Indeed, I have intended to explore how the values of American culture, the institutional arrangements of the society as a whole and of the field of medicine in particular, have created a particular milieu which significantly influences the lives of dying individuals. In a certain sense, formulating the question of modern dying in terms of its dimensions as a public issue contains an ultimate irony. The more the troubles of dying individuals are framed by isolation, psychologizing, and privatization, the more these processes of individuation reflect a collective drift and pattern of modern death. In this way, the tendency to define and isolate each individual's death in a private world of coping is itself a manifestation of a public issue. Thus, the more dying and its psychological ameliorations are encapsulated in the framework of private troubles, the more this situation itself is a public issue worthy of study.

The result of my application of Mills' sociological imagination is a portrait of the modern dying patient as perceived from an admittedly critical viewpoint. Just as a landscape or portrait which takes form on a painter's canvas reflects the special viewpoint of the painter, sociological portraits necessarily reflect the viewpoint of the sociological artist, that is to say, they have been transmuted and filtered through the artist's perception, consciousness, and style [2, p. 42].

Nisbet, in his classic book, *Sociology As An Art Form*, discusses the role of art within the discipline and defines artistic sociology not as a fleeting fad but as being very much anchored in the classicism and historical traditions of the field:

> Far from least among sociology's contributions in the nineteenth century is the distinctive ways in which its practitioners saw the landscape in human affairs that had been so largely created by the two great revolutions ... Not quantitative, empirical science following any of the contrived prescriptions of current textbooks in methodology or theory construction, but the artist's vision, lies behind such concepts as mass society, Gemeinschaft, Gesellschaft, social status, authority, the sacred and the secular, alienation, anomie, and the other signal reactions to the European social landscape in the nineteenth century that we properly associate with the development of sociology [2, p. 43].

I have sought in *On Death Without Dignity: The Human Impact of Technological Dying* to paint an iconic portrait of the human experience of dying in the modern, medicalized social setting. In painting a portrait of modern dying, the real life experiences of dying patients were essential to shaping and framing my portrayal of the modern dying experience. It was therefore essential for me to enter into the backrooms of medicine, where I could observe and study the life circumstances of hospitalized, dying patients as unobtrusively as possible, and to get as close to the life circumstances of these dying patients as I possibly could.

In adopting the strategies for observational research as set forth in the *Discovery of Grounded Theory* [6] and *Field Research: Strategies for a Natural Sociology* [7], observation and interviews were the two dominant mechanisms of accumulating a body of research materials on the human process of dying. The research materials were gathered at an urban medical center with a strong teaching emphasis. I gained entrance into the professional and personal worlds of dying, which are formed in the medical center, by associating myself with a faculty-oncologist who was receptive to the goals of my research plan. During the four-month exploratory phase of the study, I accompanied him on his daily rounds. This enabled me to begin to see patients every day and to establish a sense of normalcy to my presence in the medical setting. It also provided the opportunity to begin to establish a sense of ease and comfort with patients, whom I would see at moments of great physical and emotional vulnerability. The development of this sense of faith and trust in me was essential to getting as close as possible to the world of dying patients, and was something that slowly developed. Once this basis of trust was achieved, the openness with which patients spoke to me and their lack of concern with maintaining behavorial appearances in front of me was rather striking. The painfully honest sentiments which are reflected by the words of the dying contained in this book are an indicator of the trust that I established with these patients.

During the fourteen months which constituted the main body of fieldwork, I spent my time on rounds, observing, listening, and talking to dying patients. My observations led me to witness the following situations and/or settings: physicians talking to each other in hallways, elevators, and stairwells about medical or non-medical matters; physicians formally and informally consulting about specific cases; patients being examined; patients relating to family members; physicians discussing x-rays and other test results; nurses and doctors relating to each other; and interns relating to attending physicians. By being able to integrate into the backrooms of medicine, two salient advantages occurred. First, I was able to see what the physician sees but the patient does not. For example, I saw, discussed, and was taught about the medical condition of each of the patients in the study through their x-rays. I was thus able to see the biological-technological underpinnings of physician activity, which take place in the backrooms of the hospital setting. Second, by spending time each day with patients, while they were admitted in the hospital, I was able to integrate into the human concerns and world view of dying patients and their families. I was, therefore, the beneficiary of seeing and being a part of the human process of dying, from which physicians and other medical caretakers are isolated. This double perspective on dying enabled me to look at the process of dying through the frame of reference of both physicians and dying patients.

Thirty-seven patients were in the study. Nineteen of them were male, with an age range from twenty-two to ninety. All of the patients in the study were in the advanced stages of cancer, i.e., they were at post-surgical and radiation treatment stages, and were subjectively defined by their attending oncologist as having potentially fatal disease and only months to live. Some patients lingered on for unexpectedly long periods of time, while others died rather quickly— but all of them now are dead.

I do not mean to imply that dying from cancer in a major, urban medical center is the only way of dying in American society. Clearly, people die from other chronic diseases and/or medical circumstances. Moreover, people die in nursing homes, community hospitals, hospices, and at home. But, first of all, cancer does provide a model disease for studying the modern processes of dying in that it represents a chronic illness trajectory, which increasingly typifies modern illness and dying. Also, the cultural meanings of cancer, so nicely portrayed by Sontag's *Illness As Metaphor* [8] , are such that the deepest fears and terrors of modern people, with regard to dying and death, are embodied in the human cancer experience. Second, I have elected to study dying in the setting of the urban medical center precisely because that environment is reflective of the most modern style of dying found in American society today. Thus, I have sought to create and portray an impression of dying in America that reflects the cultural and social drift toward modernity. I do not mean to imply, however, that variations of dying styles are not possible or do not occur within the modern framework.

A final methodological note is worth mentioning. The sensitivity of the topic of dying, its deeply personal implications, and the fact that I would regularly see patients during times of heightened vulnerability, helped to create a special and complex role for me in the lives of the dying patients who participated in the study. There was a tendency on the part of the patients to begin to see me not only as a researcher but also as a source of support—someone who would offer comfort during times of emotional turmoil, someone they would generally see daily during the course of their hospital stay, someone they could complain to, etc. Indeed, the more open and painfully honest patients were in their conversations with me, the more they identified me as being more than just a socio-medical researcher.

While the issue of establishing workable, amicable relationships with the people one is studying is critical in all types of naturalistic sociological research, the circumstances of dying and death make the development of such relationships and their implications for all involved, all the more notable. In order to penetrate into the worlds and sub-worlds of dying patients, I found it essential to get close to the lives of dying patients. The result was that I became a part of their lives. Although it is beyond my intent to write on the dilemmas of naturalistic research with dying people, the role of such research in the lives of the dying and the way in which the study of the process of dying creates special consequences for naturalistic fieldwork are important topics worthy of future consideration. But I can say this: The complexities, vulnerabilities, and deeply private nature of modern dying require a very special humanistic connection between researcher and participant, if the study is to succeed in penetrating into and portraying the deeply hidden human dimensions of dying and death.

One of the cornerstones of successful social science research is that the people who are being studied will recognize themselves in the written account of the study [6, 9]. If dying patients and their intimates can see themselves in my portrait, I will have been successful in capturing the systems of meaning and the world view of the dying patients themselves. If physicians who regularly work with dying patients can divorce themselves from their own professional world view and see some of the human consequences of medicalized dying, I will have succeeded. Additionally, if you, the reader, have been touched by this portrait of dying or have found that it provoked thought, reflection, or insight, I will have been successful in debunking and portraying the human and social implications of modern dying. In this way, the humanistic-sociomedical study of dying and death may not be fully value-free, but it is always value-relevant.

REFERENCES

1. A. Giddens, *Sociology: A Brief but Critical Introduction*. Harcourt, Brace, Jovanovich, New York, 1982.
2. R. Nisbet, *Sociology as an Art Form*, Oxford University Press, New York, 1977.
3. C. Bosk, The Fieldworker as Watcher and Witness, *The Hastings Center Report 15*:3, 1985.
4. P. Berger, *Invitation to Sociology*, Doubleday and Co., New York, 1963.
5. C. W. Mills, *The Sociological Imagination*, Oxford University Press, New York, 1959.
6. B. Glaser and A. Strauss, *Discovery of Grounded Theory: Strategies for Qualitative Research*, Aldine Publishing Co., Chicago, 1967.
7. L. Schatzman and A. Strauss, *Field Research: Strategies for a Natural Sociology*, Prentice-Hall, New Jersey, 1973.
8. S. Sontag, *Illness As Metaphor*, Vintage Books, New York, 1979.
9. A. Strauss et al., *Social Organization of Medical Work*, University of Chicago Press, 1985. See the Preface and Methodological Appendix.

Index

Watts School of Nursing Library
D.C.H.C.

Watts School of Nursing Library
D.C.H.C.

DATE DUE

DATE DUE			
APR. 4 '94			
JUN 8 '95			
10-17-96			
NOV 12			
NOV 5 1998			
MAR 3 0 1999			
APR 2 0 1999			
GAYLORD			PRINTED IN U.S.A.